Royal Society of Medicine

International Congress and Symposium Series

Number 14

The Cardiovascular, Metabolic and Psychological Interface

Condensed proceedings of a Symposium organized by CIBA and supported by the International Society and Federation of Cardiology, on 1–3 December, 1978, at the Hilton Hotel, Stratford-upon-Avon.

Royal Society of Medicine

International Congress and Symposium Series

Number 14

The Cardiovascular, Metabolic and Psychological Interface

Edited by

R. W. ELSDON-DEW, C. A. S. WINK and G. F. B. BIRDWOOD

1979

Published jointly by

THE ROYAL SOCIETY OF MEDICINE
1 Wimpole Street, London

ACADEMIC PRESS
London

GRUNE & STRATTON
New York

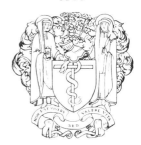

ROYAL SOCIETY OF MEDICINE
1 Wimpole Street, London W1M 8AE

ACADEMIC PRESS INC. (LONDON) LTD.
24/28 Oval Road, London NW1 7DX

United States Edition published and distributed by

GRUNE & STRATTON INC.
111 Fifth Avenue, New York, New York 10013

Copyright © 1979 by

ROYAL SOCIETY OF MEDICINE and
ACADEMIC PRESS INC. (LONDON) LTD.

The cardiovascular, metabolic and psychological interface.—(Royal Society of Medicine. International congress and symposium series; no. 14 ISSN 0142-2367).
1. Cardiovascular system—Diseases—Congresses
2. Cardiovascular system—Diseases—Psychosomatic aspects—Congresses
3. Psychology, Physiological—Congresses I. Elsdon-Dew, R. W. II. Wink, Charles Anthony Stewart. III. Birdwood, George Fortune Broderick. IV. Series
616.1'08   RC669   79-40098

ISBN (Academic Press): 0-12-791155-3

ISBN (Grune & Stratton): 0-8089-1219-4

Printed in Great Britain by Spottiswoode Ballantyne Ltd., Colchester and London.

Contributors

Speakers

P. W. Adams	*St Mary's Hospital, London*
L. C. Antal	*Cressington Park, Liverpool*
P. Biggs	*Walsgrave Hospital, Coventry*
M. Carruthers	*The Maudsley Hospital, London*
G. E. Foster	*Nottingham General Hospital, Nottingham*
C. W. H. Havard	*Royal Northern Hospital, London*
J. R. Hawkings	*Sedgefield, Stockton-on-Tees, Cleveland*
B. I. Hoffbrand	*Whittington Hospital, London*
H. Keen	*Guy's Hospital, London*
M. Lader	*Institute of Psychiatry, London*
A. H. Mann	*Institute of Psychiatry, London*
D. R. Master	*Institute of Psychiatry, London*
I. Mills	*Addenbrooke's Hospital, Cambridge*
R. Rosenman	*Harold Brunn Institute, San Francisco*
P. S. Sever	*St Mary's Hospital, London*
M. R. Stephens	*University Hospital of Wales, Cardiff*
S. H. Taylor	*Leeds General Infirmary, Leeds*
T. Theorell	*Huddinge University Hospital, Sweden*

Chairmen

I. H. Mills	*Addenbrookes Hospital, Cambridge*
R. Rosenman	*Harold Brunn Institute, San Francisco*
S. H. Taylor	*Leeds General Infirmary, Leeds*

Contents

Section ID : Metabolic Responses

Section II : The Metabolic and Cardiovascular Connection

Section III : The Psychological and Cardiovascular Connection

Preface

Medicine today has become highly technical and, as a result, doctors have had to become more and more specialized. Few hospital consultants now are broad specialists in the way that general physicians used to be—though the term itself still persists. Most are now well on the way to becoming sub-specialists in parts of their chosen field.

This degree of specialization may obscure the interaction between the different systems and sub-systems that make up man—and medicine—as a whole. It is therefore vital that physicians and research workers with specialized knowledge in differing yet interrelated areas of medicine should meet to exchange views.

Cardiovascular morbidity is a case in point. Understanding of its causation depends—among other things—on knowledge of the interactions between psychological, social and metabolic changes. Furthermore, treatment apparently directed at one or other aspect of these changes may affect the others. The symposium reported here was designed to facilitate interdisciplinary discussion in this field—with the ultimately practical aim of promoting further advances in the prophylaxis and therapy of cardiovascular disease.

The Editors

Emotions, Physiology and Stress
(Abstract)

M. LADER

Institute of Psychiatry, University of London

Emotion can be regarded as an introspective experience, a *noumenon*. As such it is an irreducible concept, not susceptible to scientific analysis. Emotion can also be considered as a verbal report of the subjective state which can be analysed and quantified. However, the relationship between verbal report (i.e. speech) and emotion (i.e. feeling) remains unvalidated.

and from the psychiatrist in the outpatients clinic. It can be excessive in two ways: quantitatively, as in the case of clinical anxiety, which is an emotion too severe, too persistent or too pervasive for the patient to tolerate (that is, quantitatively abnormal in degree, time or space); and qualitatively, as in clinical depression, which differs in its quality from normal sadness. Patients can describe

Table I
Some characteristic symptoms of anxiety

Choking	Irritability	Vomiting
Smothering	Weakness	Mucous diarrhoea
Difficulty in breathing	Lump in throat	Loss of appetite
Palpitations	Overbreathing	Loss of weight
Chest pain	Pins and needles	Fear of dying
Dizziness	Repeated swallowing	Sense of insecurity
Faintness	Desire to micturate or defaecate	Fear of cancer
Fatigue	Nausea	Depersonalization

Sets of signs and symptoms (Table 1) are associated with the various emotions and may perhaps form characteristic patterns of physiological response. Overt, observable behaviours can be related to emotions. Facial expressions are the most informative of these but body posture and gait are also important. Also, emotions may interfere with or facilitate various tasks, but this action is too complex to allow for easy interpretation.

Intuitive clinical observation utilizes several of the above objective aspects but remains as unquantifiable as the subjective feeling itself. Very subtle cues such as speech content and gesture probably operate here.

When a patient's emotion becomes excessive, help may be sought from the general practitioner

the ineffable attributes of deep depression. Ecstasy is probably also outside normal experience even of euphoria.

An interesting and relevant topic is the specific patterning of physiological responses. It has been suggested that this specificity can take several forms. The pattern may, for instance, be stimulus-specific, as with penile erection related to sexual stimuli. Or it may be emotion-specific, that is, the pattern follows the type of emotion experienced by the individual. There have been surprisingly few studies in this field but it is known that anxiety is accompanied by a different pattern from that of anger. For example, blood-pressure rises are greater in anger than in anxiety but increase in heart rate is less marked. The pattern of physiological responses may also be specific for the

The Cardiovascular, Metabolic and Psychological Interface: Royal Society of Medicine International Congress and Symposium Series No. 14, published jointly by Academic Press Inc. (London) Ltd., and the Royal Society of Medicine.

personality; certain personality types may tend to respond with particular physiological changes. This theory held some vogue in psychosomatic medicine but is now largely discredited. Individual specificity may also operate: it has been suggested that each individual has an idiosyncratic pattern of response. The style of response—how the subject reacts to the stimulus—has also to be taken into account. For example, if he defends against a loud noise, heart rate rises: this would be his "defensive reflex". If he responds or "orients" himself towards a less loud noise, heart rate drops as part of the "orienting" or "what-is-it?" reflex.

Selye defines stress as "the non-specific response of the body to any demand made upon it". It is immaterial whether the demand is pleasant or unpleasant. This definition is probably too wide-ranging to be meaningful. Both "non-specific" and "demand" are awkward terms, the latter especially containing the germs of tautology. Stress is the body's response to demands, but demands can only be defined in terms of producing stress. Thus, a scientific concept of the 1930s

misnamed but still definable in terms of tissue changes has lost scientific credibility. We should concentrate on stimulus–response relationships with careful study of the physiological changes accompanying the behaviour responses (see Fig. 1). The term "stress" is relegated to a convenient non-technical shorthand term which communicates our ignorance, not our knowledge.

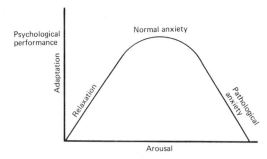

Figure 1. Psychological performance is improved up to a certain point by arousal, but then falls off.

Discussion

P. G. F. Nixon

I was surprised that you did not discuss the subject of habituation. In the cardio-vascular field, our clinical observations of angina, hypertension and arrhythmias suggest that highly aroused and exhausted patients respond as if they cannot habituate to some of the important sources of arousal around them. This seems to be a more important cause of severe sympatho-adrenal overactivity than simple elevation of the circulating catecholamines.

M. Lader

I mentioned adaptation at the end and include habituation under that heading— adaptation being a change in the tonic, background response level, and habituation a decrement over repeated responses. When the arousal level gets too high, one impairment of function is the inability to adapt and/or habituate to external stimulation (see Fig. 1). Indeed, under certain circumstances of high arousal, in contrast to habituation, the responses get larger and larger. It is very difficult to know whether arousal is high because habituation takes place slowly or fails in high arousal states. There might even be a positive feedback loop, but I know of no feasible way of studying such a system in the laboratory.

P. G. F. Nixon

It is very important that light should be thrown upon habituation, because it is usually assumed that people with "hypertension" have high catecholamine levels— and the condition should be diagnosable from the blood or urine concentrations. Habituation is a much more satisfactory theory because it does not demand high catecholamine levels in hypertension, and because it can explain the changing patterns in people who shift into and out of phases of hypertension and homoeostasis violation as their arousal rises to morbid levels and falls again.

G. H. Hall

To what extent do these responses have to be learned? I can remember vividly my elementary school teacher giving me hell over mental arithmetic, and I imagine that is why I still get arousal responses now. On the other hand, a child playing with fire does not get aroused because he has not learned what it means.

M. Lader

Certainly association of the verbal report—what the subject says he is feeling—with the feeling itself has to be learned. Patients may use the wrong words. When psychiatric patients complaining of depression or anxiety are asked to explain what they are feeling, they often misuse words describing emotion, presumably because they have learned little expertise in word-usage. Moreover, if there is an appreciable physiological response to anxiety, the subject learns to associate his subjective feelings with the physiological changes. Palpitations, for instance, may generate an expectation of anxiety. Some of the differences observed with infusion of catecholamines may be because patients associate the resulting palpitations with anxiety, whereas normal subjects have not learned such an association.

V. Hrubes

In the past there has been much misunderstanding of the word "stress", which is commonly used to describe both the cause and the syndrome of reactions, i.e. the response. Lately the term "stressor" has been employed for the cause.

M. Lader

We have to accept that "stress" is now used mainly to describe the response. We should avoid using it for the external stimulus as well—the "stressor". However, we assume that any powerful stimulation must be a "stress", and that any "stress" response must be the result of such stimulation. We could with advantage avoid the term entirely and speak of stimulus and response.

R. Rosenman

Considering the dramatic differences in feelings between, say anger and ecstasy, can we really believe that measurement by venous plethysmography in the arm accurately measures these differences?

M. Lader

One measurement gives some idea of the general level of emotional intensity, but no information about its nature. For that we have to rely on observation, facial expression and asking the subjects themselves. Even with a whole pattern of responses, we cannot say which emotion the person is feeling. However, if we induce two different emotions in one subject, we can guess to some extent which of the two he is feeling by the particular pattern of responses.

Life Events and Ischaemic Heart Disease
(Abstract)

T. THEORELL

*Institute of Social Medicine,
Huddinge University Hospital, Sweden*

Psychosocial factors may contribute to the development of clinical coronary heart disease in several ways: by accelerating atherosclerosis through "voluntary" acts such as cigarette smoking, wrong diet and lack of exercise, which are known to be risk factors and via neuro-hormonal pathways affecting blood pressure, lipid metabolism and coagulation mechanisms; and also by suddenly upsetting cardiovascular equilibrium, thereby "precipitating" acute episodes of coronary heart disease.

Such episodes may be precipitated instantaneously, as in the case of life-threatening disturbances of cardiac rhythm, or be delayed; indeed, there is no clear distinction between predisposing and precipitating mechanisms. Furthermore, internal (constitutional or hereditary) and external (social and environmental) factors interact. It is thus not possible to separate the influence of life events from that of the wide array of other factors playing an important part in causing clinical manifestations of coronary heart disease.

Genetic Studies in Twins

The potential importance of genetic factors was shown (Fig. 1) in a study of heart rate, systolic and diastolic blood pressure and pulse volume in 17 pairs of male monozygotic twins and 13 pairs of male dizygotic twins aged 52–74 years (Theorell *et al.*, 1979). Within-pairs variance in these factors during a psychiatric interview was significantly less in monozygotic than in dizygotic twins. Heart rate was the only variable in which within-pairs variance was significantly smaller in mono-

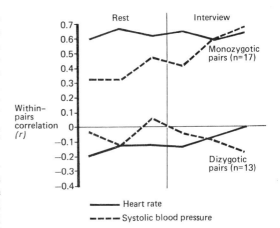

Figure 1. Blood pressure and heart rate responses in monozygotic and dizygotic twins.

zygotic than in dizygotic twins both at rest and during interview: in the case of the other variables, a significant effect of genetic influence was observed only during interview. For example, during rest the within-pairs correlation r for systolic blood pressure was about 0·3, whereas at the end of the interview r = 0·68. One possible interpretation of this observation is that genetic factors are more important when the response provoked is a primitive one: this may be particularly the case when the response is peripheral vasoconstriction and elevation of the blood pressure. Excessive, repeated, acute reactions of this kind may form the basis for neurogenic hypertension.

The Cardiovascular, Metabolic and Psychological Interface: Royal Society of Medicine International Congress and Symposium Series No. 14, published jointly by Academic Press Inc. (London) Ltd., and the Royal Society of Medicine.

Identification of Psychosocial Pressures

A number of retrospective and prospective studies have been carried out to determine precisely which psychosocial pressures are most commonly present before the onset of myocardial infarction or sudden coronary death, and which are found significantly more frequently than expected. In Sweden it has been a consistent finding that, in the year preceding myocardial infarction, pressures at work (changes in responsibility, excessive responsibility, conflicts and extra work) have been reported more often than would be expected, while financial and family pressures have not been so strikingly associated. However, in a recent comparative study of Americans and Swedes with and without clinical evidence of coronary heart disease (Orth-Gomér, 1979), family pressures but not work pressures were strongly associated in the American subjects with onset of clinically overt coronary heart disease, while in the Swedish subjects the expected association with work pressures was found. Marked cultural differences may therefore account for some of the disparate findings in this field (for noradrenaline studies see Fig. 2).

Value of Recording Life Events

According to Holmes and Rahe (1967), "life change measurement" is not an accurate predictor of myocardial infarction. But at the Huddinge

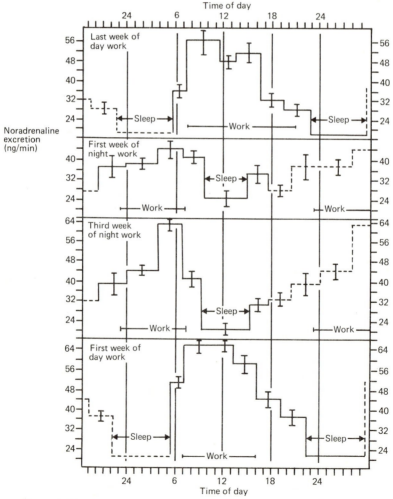

Figure 2. Noradrenaline excretion under different conditions of shift work.

Hospital we find it very useful in the clinical setting to record events occurring in the patient's life shortly before onset of disease, and patients too find it helpful to discuss them. Also a long-term follow-up study has shown that in most patients rehabilitated after myocardial infarction such events may predict rises in catecholamine output which are potentially important for pathophysiology.

Finally, acute psychosocial problems which have arisen during the year before onset of disease may markedly influence the psychological component of the illness during the patient's stay in hospital.

References

Holmes, T. H. and Rahe, R. H. (1967). The social readjustment rating scale. *J. psychosom. Res.* **17**, 213.

Orth-Gomér, K. (1979). Ischaemic heart disease and psychological stress in Stockholm and New York. *J. psychosom. Res.* (in press).

Theorell, T., Schalling, D., de Faire, U., Adamson, U. and Askevold, F. (1979). Personality traits and psychophysiological reactions to a stressful interview in twins with varying degrees of coronary heart disease. *J. psychosom. Res.* (in press).

Further Reading

Theorell, T. and Floderus-Myrhed, B. (1977). Workload and risk of myocardial infarction—a prospective psychosocial analysis. *Int. J. Epidem.* **6**, 17.

Theorell, T. *et al.* (1975). The relationship of disturbing life-changes and emotions to the early development of myocardial infarction and other serious illnesses. *Int. J. Epidem.* **4**, 291.

Discussion

E. Jackson

If we are to believe that there is a pre-infarction syndrome, and we must all be familiar with some patients feeling unwell for a time before they have an infarct, surely work stress is going to show itself at that stage because a previously well-adapted man is already becoming poorly adapted. Would this not be a possible explanation of your finding that work stress is the factor most closely related to future infarction?

T. Theorell

It is always difficult to sort out such possibilities. But the way these people describe their situations has convinced me that we are dealing with something which starts in the environment, affects the physiology and then interacts with it. From the epidemiological viewpoint, I see the apparent emphasis on work stress as unimportant because we are dealing with a syndrome. If this can be identified months before the infarction then possibly something could be done to reduce the degree of risk— and reducing work stress would obviously be one candidate for prophylactic action, whatever its precise role. In the follow-up of myocardial infarction, we exclude those who had been absent from work because of heart disease, hypertension or diabetes during the year preceding follow-up; but still included those with a previous history of chest pain who developed myocardial infarction during the 2-year follow-up. If the latter were excluded, the association between the psychosocial workload and the risk of myocardial infarction was still significant, ($P < 0.01$) and even increased somewhat—48% reporting psychosocial work stress, against 25% expected, after correction for age. The corresponding numbers before exclusion of those with a previous history of chest pain were 37% and 23%.

E. Jackson

The main point of your paper seemed to be that psychosocial factors could lead on to physical disease, but the alternative theory—that physical factors might lead to psychosocial distress seemed equally likely.

T. Theorell

In this study the subjects all did heavy manual work, which makes it very unlikely that they would have had cardiovascular pathophysiological symptoms.

H. Keen

To what extent do you think the answers to the questions you are asking may be determined by the way that you are asking them? That is to say, if you confront people with a list of "dysgratifying" or unpleasant events, and accept ordinary statistical probability levels, the likelihood of chance association between them is quite large. If you ask twenty questions, then one in twenty is likely to come up positive, and one in twenty negative. Did you provide alternative options by asking about the good things that happened in life—could it be that ecstasy is a forerunner of ischaemic heart disease?

T. Theorell

The danger of asking so many questions that some would be likely to achieve statistical significance anyway was excluded by the way we constructed the trial protocol. As regards work stress, we formulated a hypothesis that a cluster of items would be associated with increased risk of infarction and designed the study to test that specific association.

Hypertension and the Environment
(Extended Abstract)

P. S. SEVER

St Mary's Hospital Medical School, London

Blood Pressure, Age and Way of Life

The bushmen of the Kalahari desert migrated into southern Africa over 1000 years ago but only 25,000 of them survive today, many having remained essentially nomadic and surviving by hunting and scavenging for food. To epidemiologists they remain of considerable interest for they form one of the few populations in whom blood pressure (Fig. 1) does not rise with age (Truswell *et al.*, 1972). The Negro Africans or Bantu differ strikingly from the bushmen, being offshoots of central African Negro stock that migrated southwards and westwards over many centuries.

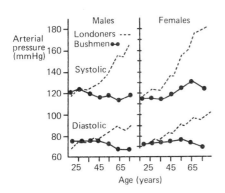

Figure 1. Blood pressure does not necessarily rise with age (from Truswell et al., *1972).*

Even today the tribal and more primitive Africans appear to share with the bushmen an environment which permits blood pressure to rise little with advancing age (Scotch, 1963). On the other hand,

when the Bantu tribesman migrates from tribe to township, a different pattern emerges: his blood pressure rises dramatically with age (Fig. 2) and he suffers from the consequences of such elevated pressures, with cardiac failure, stroke and renal disease. In this he resembles the North American and West Indian Negro and indeed shows the blood-pressure/age relationship seen in Caucasian communities.

However, in some epidemiological studies of blood pressure in rural and urban populations, no clear-cut differences have been found. In West Indians, for example, blood pressure was found to rise with age in both rural and urban populations (Miall *et al.*, 1962). On the other hand the "rural" West Indian is far removed culturally and socio-economically from the tribesmen of the Transkei and has experienced at least some of the consequences of "Westernization".

There is a wealth of data on the way in which blood pressure varies with age in different black communities. Epstein and Eckhoff (1967) found that the blood pressures of African, Caribbean and North American Negroes tended not to rise with age in nomadic and rural populations, but did so markedly in the USA and in urban black communities.

Such changes in arterial pressures are not confined to Negro populations. Beaglehole *et al.* (1977) followed up a population of south-sea-island dwellers (the Tokelauans) during their migration to New Zealand and their subsequent integration into New Zealand society. Again it was found that higher blood pressures developed following migration in certain groups.

If migration from one environment to another results in an elevation in blood pressure in some

The Cardiovascular, Metabolic and Psychological Interface: Royal Society of Medicine International Congress and Symposium Series No. 14, published jointly by Academic Press Inc. (London) Ltd., and the Royal Society of Medicine.

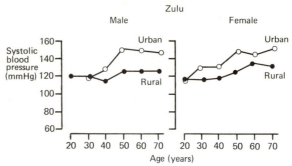

Figure 2. Among urban dwellers blood pressure does tend to rise with age irrespective of race (from Scotch, 1963).

communities, what factor or factors may be involved, and how may urbanization or acculturation influence arterial pressure? Dietary change and "stress" appear to be important.

Salt and Hypertension

Of many dietary constituents, salt has generated the most interest and its relation to blood pressure has been debated for several decades. Prehistoric man was a sodium-deficient herbivore, and all the available evidence suggests that twentieth-century Westernized man consumes far in excess of his metabolic needs, which can be sustained on a modest 1–2 g/day (Fig. 3).

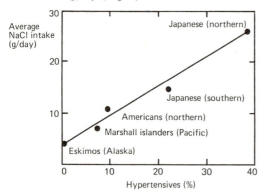

Figure 3. Sodium chloride intake in excess of metabolic needs is directly associated with hypertension, regardless of race (from Dahl, 1961).

In Robert Burton's seventeenth-century treatise *The Anatomy of Melancholy*, the author considered salt and salt meats to be great procurers of the disease. The writings on the evils of salt have, however, much older origins: the priests of Ancient Egypt abstained from salt "so that their souls would be free from perturbations".

In the classic experiments of Meneely *et al.* (1953), diets containing salt in various quantities

were fed to rats over a 9-month period; frank hypertension with morbidity and premature death occurred in those rats on a high-salt diet, but to a lesser extent when the diet was rich in potassium. Epidemiological studies followed and, in summary, confirmed that populations consuming diets containing less than 2 g/day of salt have low blood pressures that fail to rise with age.

Prior and Evans (1969) studied New Guinea natives, who take a low-salt diet, but blood pressures rose and hypertension occurred when such people moved to modern coastal cities where dietary salt was much higher. The bushmen's diet also is low in salt which is in line with their low blood pressures. At the other extreme, high salt intakes are associated with a high prevalence of hypertension, as for example in Japanese farmers who consume up to 35 g/day (Fig. 3).

Preliminary data from our own investigations reveal much lower dietary salt and urinary sodium excretion in Transkei villagers than in the urban communities where hypertension is more common. Finally, in two Polynesian island groups investigated by Prior *et al.* (1968), similar in most respects, the higher pressures in one island community related to a very much higher dietary sodium intake.

However, some individuals can take huge amounts of salt without its affecting their blood pressure, while in others arterial pressure will be markedly raised. Dahl (1961) proposed that individual responses to salt may be genetically determined—a factor seemingly confirmed in his ability to breed out from a single strain of rats one substrain which was salt-sensitive and another which was salt-resistant. In the latter a rise in cardiac output, together with a fall in total peripheral vascular resistance, occurred early on; both functions returned to normal after 1 week of salt loading and blood pressure remained unchanged. In the salt-sensitive rats, the early rise in cardiac output was associated with a rise in peripheral vascular resistance and an elevation of arterial pressure; following salt loading for 1 week, cardiac output returned to normal, but a further rise in peripheral vascular resistance occurred and the blood pressure rose further.

The vascular response to sodium, which may be genetically determined, could therefore be the factor which controls whether or not blood pressure will rise.

Physical and Emotional Stress, and Hypertension

When populations migrate, individuals find themselves in totally strange environments to which they must adjust, and the process of urbanization or acculturation may exert major effects upon the human subject and his cardiovascular system. The role of psychosocial stress in the elevation of blood pressure remains an interesting hypothesis, but one for which hard evidence is difficult to obtain, at least in man.

In Beaglehole's study of blood pressure and social interaction among Tokelauan migrants in New Zealand (1977), an interaction index was derived by assessing the extent to which each of 635 adult Tokelauans integrated into New Zealand society, as judged by ethnic affiliation of workmates and friends, club membership, whether or not they participated in Tokelauan community and religious activities (Tokelauan or New Zealand), language fluency and so on. The greater the interaction with New Zealand society, the higher was the arterial pressure found to be.

To determine how far this rise in blood pressure is due to stress is a difficult but nevertheless interesting problem to study. From experiments in animals it seems likely that the central nervous system may play an important role in elevating the blood pressure in particular behavioural situations. Exaggerated pressure rises in response to stress have been observed in some animals, notably the "spontaneous hypertensive" rat, and it has been suggested that in this species even normal environmental stimuli may interact with an inherent hyper-reactivity of the defence mechanism—and that the more frequent and powerful neurogenic pressure rises contribute to the development of hypertension. It is noteworthy that isolated animals of the same species, removed from such stimuli at the time of weaning, have much lower pressures.

Physical and emotional stress exert profound effects through the autonomic nervous system, and activation of the sympatho-adrenal system in animals and man results in markedly elevated levels of circulating catecholamines. Such changes

in sympathetic activity are generally of limited duration, but in the case of repeated emotional stress there is evidence for a more prolonged effect on the integrity of the system, in that the activity of the catecholamine biosynthetic enzymes is increased through the hypothalamic–pituitary–adrenal axis.

The case in man for increased sympathetic activity in essential hypertension is far from being established. Nevertheless, there is evidence that haemodynamic responses to physical stresses may be excessive in some hypertensive subjects during the early stages of the blood pressure rise; and the consensus is that the circulating catecholamines, particularly following physical stresses, are raised in this group of patients. Data on the effects of emotional stimuli are limited; nevertheless, it is tempting to suggest that over-reactivity to everyday stress could lead to established hypertension. Until we have better methods of measuring stress and its various effects upon the circulation, the problem will remain unanswered.

Our own studies strongly suggest differences between races in this respect. To date we have found no evidence for excessive sympathetic responses in blacks and the only abnormality identified is that occurring in young white subjects with essential hypertension, in whom high resting circulating catecholamine levels are found and excessive responses occur with physical stress (Sever *et al.*, 1978).

My present (by no means original) view is that certain environmental factors can elevate arterial pressure: dietary sodium through its effects on extracellular fluid volume; stress through activation of the autonomic nervous system. However, it requires a genetically determined predisposition before such individuals respond to their environmental insult with sustained elevation of blood pressure.

I also believe that the relative importance of differing environmental and genetic factors may vary from individual to individual and between different ethnic groups. One has only to view some of the characteristics of essential hypertension in the black to arrive at the conclusion that it is a very different condition from that seen in the white, and therefore perhaps due to different pathogenetic mechanisms.

We are in the early stages of studying further differences between blacks and whites with respect to their blood pressures in different environments, in the hope that new light may be shed upon the relative contributions of genetic and environmental factors in the development of human essential hypertension.

References

Beaglehole, R., Salmond, C. E., Hooper, A., Huntsman, J., Stanhope, J. M., Cassel, J. C. and Prior, I. A. M. (1977). Blood pressure and social interaction in Tokelauan migrants in New Zealand. *J. chron. Dis.* **30,** 803–812.

Dahl, L. K. (1961). Possible role of chronic excess salt consumption in the pathogenesis of essential hypertension. *Amer. J. Cardiol.* **8,** 571–575.

Epstein, F. H. and Eckhoff, R. D. (1967). The epidemiology of high blood pressure. *In* "The Epidemiology of Hypertension: Proceedings of an International Symposium" (Ed. Stamler, J., Stamler, R. and Pullman, T. N.), p. 155. Grune & Stratton, New York.

Meneely, G. R., Tucker, R. G., Darby, W. J. and Auerbach, S. D. (1953). Chronic sodium chloride toxicity in albino rat. II. Occurrence of hypertension and of syndrome of oedema and renal failure. *J. exp. Med.* **98,** 71.

Miall, W. E., Kass, E. H., Ling, J. and Stuart, K. L. (1962). Factors influencing arterial pressure in the general population of Jamaica. *Brit. med. J.* **2,** 497.

Prior, I. A. M. and Evans, J. G. (1969). Sodium intake and blood pressure in Pacific populations. *Israel J. med. Sci.* **5,** 609.

Prior, I. A. M., Grimley-Evans, J., Harvey, H. P. B., Davidson, F. and Lindsey, M. (1968). Sodium intake and blood pressure in two Polynesian populations. *New Engl. J. Med.* **279,** 515–520.

Scotch, N. A. (1963). Sociocultural factors in the epidemiology of Zulu hypertension *Amer. J. publ. Hlth.* **53,** 1205–1213.

Sever, P. S., Peart, W. S., Meade, T., Davies, I. B., Gordon, D. and Tunbridge, R. D. G. (1978). Are racial differences in essential hypertension due to different pathogenetic mechanisms? *Clin. Sci. molec. Med.* **55** (Suppl. 4), 383s–389s.

Truswell, A. S., Kennelly, B. M., Hansen, J. D. L. and Lee, R. B. (1972). Blood pressure of !Kung bushmen in Northern Botswana. *Amer. Heart J.* **84,** 5–12.

Discussion

I. H. Mills

In many of the groups of individuals or animals that you have discussed, there is a physiological factor which plays a very big part in determining sensitivity to factors promoting hypertension. This physiological factor is the enzyme kallikrein, which releases bradykinin—a very potent vasodilator. It has been shown by workers in the United States and Nigeria that the black races have very low urinary kallikrein excretion. Kallikrein in the urine comes entirely from the kidney, and we have found that kallikrein released from the kidney also enters the general circulation and almost certainly plays a part in lowering blood pressure. In blacks, kallikrein excretion is not affected by blood pressure level but in whites it is much higher in normotensives. When essential hypertension develops in whites their kallikrein level drops to that seen in blacks. In animals, Dahl's salt-sensitive rats all have low kallikrein excretion levels and salt-resistant rats have high levels. "Spontaneously hypertensive" rats after the age of three weeks have markedly lower kallikrein excretion than normotensive, related rats. So the ability to respond to stimuli by releasing kallikrein from the kidney into the circulation is probably important in determining whether the subject is hypertensive or not. In our studies, the factor obviously able to lower the release of kallikrein from the kidney is noradrenaline, or renal sympathetic nerve stimulation. I suspect that the stress effects which have been described relate to the effects of noradrenaline or sympathetic nerve drive in lowering the renal kallikrein excretion, after which the blood pressure is much less likely to stay down. From the physiological point of view, the most striking example of the importance of kallikrein is in Bartter's syndrome, in which the renin level is higher than in any other known circumstance, but so also is the kallikrein level. The two balance each other to produce normal blood pressure.

P. S. Sever

It would be very interesting if there were a change in kallikrein in black populations when they move from a primitive environment into an urban one.

I. H. Mills

Kallikrein excretion in blacks in the USA is very similar to that in Nigerians, i.e. low in both cases.

P. G. F. Nixon

Rapid urbanization is associated with a failure of homoeostasis in many functions, not only in blood pressure but diabetes, heart disease, gout and many others. If we extrapolate Dale Clark's observations in "Aviation Space and Environmental Medicine" (1975), excessive noradrenaline secretion is associated with a hard life and rises in blood uric acid with persistent anxiety. Noradrenaline levels can be related to diabetes and hypertension; is it not unfair to blame the diet for these disorders? Would it not be more reasonable to say that rapid changes in society challenge us to adapt at a rate at which we cannot maintain our homoeostasis? The principal violators of homoeostasis are excesses of noradrenaline and adrenaline, but inability to habituate to these excesses may be responsible for the defeat which brings the adrenal cortex strongly into play.

P. S. Sever

It is extremely difficult to discriminate between any possible effects of diet and those effects of urbanization which may be brought about by neurogenic mechanisms. As you pointed out, the changes in blood pressure observed in migrating populations occur very rapidly. It is not necessary to remain resident in an urban environment for, say, 30 years, before developing or becoming at risk of developing hypertension. However, this does not seem to me to distinguish between dietary and neurogenic factors, because both could change simultaneously. I am a little unhappy that all these effects should be attributed to noradrenaline and adrenaline. Although some hypertensives may have noradrenaline levels that are somewhat higher than normal, one cannot make a sweeping assertion that all hypertensives are victims of the ill-effects of noradrenaline and adrenaline—as is plain from blood determinations. Many psychiatric conditions are associated with very high levels of circulating catecholamines, and patients with these conditions are not specially prone to hypertension. Depressed patients have levels higher than those of most hypertensives.

P. G. F. Nixon

That is why I stressed the importance of habituation. Mammals which are too exhausted to habituate can show profound vascular responses to their circumstances without the blood catecholamine level changing very much. Will it not be more profitable to look at the endocrine consequences of failure to adapt quickly enough to changing circumstances, rather than restrict our attention to dietary constituents?

P. S. Sever

Yes. None of us should be so narrow-minded as to look for one particular cause. There is no single cause for hypertension; what we are seeking is an abnormal relationship between a number of factors—some environmental (in certain populations, salt may be very important) and others emotional (which may produce a major response in certain individuals). No doubt there is also interplay between the two.

G. E. Foster

Africans in towns eat less fibre than rural Africans; what part do you think dietary intake of fibre plays in blood pressure changes?

P. S. Sever

I have no idea. At this stage one can only pick out one or two possible factors for study, but I quite agree that there are many other dietary changes which should be considered—not only in fibre, but in magnesium and a whole host of elements, and other dietary factors.

C. W. H. Havard

In the savannah of Northern Nigeria, peripartum heart failure has been described in women who go into heart failure during late pregnancy or just *post partum;* this is attributed to the enormous amount of salt they take in a local potash which is believed to be good for milk production. These women do not seem to have hypertension, yet they take so much sodium that heart failure is precipitated.

P. S. Sever

Africans throughout the whole continent, and indeed in the West Indies too, very commonly develop congestive cardiomyopathy, and I am not sure whether there is any difference in the mechanism underlying peripartum cardiomyopathy and the so-called classical African cardiomyopathy. Secondly, as I said earlier, within any population there may well be a large number of subjects who do not develop hypertension even with a high-salt diet; this is evidence that more than one factor is needed: not only salt, but a particular response to that salt.

H. Keen

One environmental factor that you did not mention is fat. Most of the populations discussed grow fat as they become urbanized, particularly some of the Pacific islanders and, as I understand it, obesity has something to do with hypertension. It is certainly related to diabetes, gout and many other conditions.

P. S. Sever

I am very interested in the possibility that fatness or adiposity may be related to hypertension. The first observation that I made in Africa was the enormous difference in weight of the black women in the towns compared with the black women in the villages. The average black female whom we were seeing in the urban population weighed about 100–120 kg, whereas the average weight in village women was about 50–60 kg. However, the prevalence rates for hypertension in black females and black males are very similar; there is no great difference in weight and adiposity for black males according to where they live. This tremendous increase in weight which occurs in the urban female is not paralleled by a similar increase in the male; yet both sexes are equally liable to develop hypertension.

Reference

Clark, D. A., Arnold, E. L., Foulds, E. L. Jr., Brown, D. M., Eastmead, D. R. and Parry, E. M. (1975). Serum urate and cholesterol levels in Air Force Academy cadets. *Aviat. Space environ. Med.* **46**, 1044–1048.

Responses to Challenges of the Coping Mechanism (Abstract)

IVOR H. MILLS

Addenbrooke's Hospital, Cambridge

Using our brains is such an everyday occurrence that we rarely stop to consider if there is a limit to the number of times it can deal with challenges. Clearly a major upheaval in a person's life would be classified as stress and would impose some burden on anyone's brain. However, less severe challenges may come repeatedly. The result will be that some people will be able to cope and others will not. For those who can cope easily the demands on the brain do not impose a stress, whereas for those who cannot cope but go on trying there will be a stress response (Mills, 1976).

The frequency of challenges which can be met depends upon the length of time over which they occur. Brown and Harris (1978) have shown that most normal women can tolerate an average of 15 non-severe challenges in their lives every 3 weeks per 100 women. However, women exposed to severe events at a rate of five to ten every 3 weeks per 100 women will have a depressive breakdown if the rate suddenly rises above ten every 3 weeks.

Major challenges produce a response from the brain which resembles the "defence reaction". In animals it causes muscular vasodilatation, release of adrenaline and sympathetic nerve stimulation. In the hypothalamus there is increased release of 5-hydroxytryptamine and alteration in the control point at which cortisol (or corticosterone) can inhibit ACTH release. The result is an increase in ACTH release and adrenal stimulation. At the same time beta-lipotropin is released and converted into beta-endorphin. Elevation of 5-hydroxytryptamine in the hypothalamus also raises prolactin release and this interferes with ovulatory responses in the female.

Constant attempts to tackle challenges, either external ones or those self-generated by com-

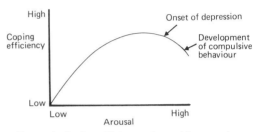

Figure 1. *Coping efficiency rises with arousal to a certain point, beyond which it falls off and gives way to depression and compulsive behaviour.*

petitive pressures, in time produces responses which lead to exhaustion of the coping process (Fig. 1). The clinical features of this include sleep disturbance, irritability, loss of appetite, menstrual disturbance, loss of libido, infertility, erectile impotence, depression, alcoholism and attempted suicide. Withdrawal from attempts to cope may prevent all these.

Raising the cerebral arousal level can facilitate coping with challenges. Commonly used stimulators are self-starvation (anorexia nervosa), caffeine, nicotine, excessively loud music, challenging the authority of parents, school teachers or the law, picking rows or fights, and self-injury with knives or by burning.

Those who have intense drive may end up with compulsive behaviour such as anorexia nervosa, compulsive eating, gambling, compulsive work, etc. When these people reach the limit of coping they are much more difficult to treat.

Excessive demand on the coping mechanism is best treated with antidepressants and these alone may play a large part in correcting endocrine disturbance.

The Cardiovascular, Metabolic and Psychological Interface: Royal Society of Medicine International Congress and Symposium Series No. 14, published jointly by Academic Press Inc. (London) Ltd., and the Royal Society of Medicine.

References

Brown, G. W. and Harris, T. (1978). "Social Origins of Depression: A study of psychiatric disorder in women." Tavistock Publications.

Mills. I. H. (1976). The disease of failure of coping. *Practitioner* **217,** 529–538.

Discussion

P. S. Sever

Data on urinary catecholamine excretion have to be interpreted with great caution. Although the changes in urinary excretion of adrenaline, noradrenaline and their metabolites which Professor Mills described in subjects shown horror films were highly significant, when compared to those seen in mild exercise they are very small. The same comparisons may be made with changes in plasma catecholamines—Dr Carruthers has shown increments of about 40–60 % when driving racing cars and speaking in public. But if changes like these are compared with those found during everyday exercise—where there may be increments of 300, 400 or even 500 %—I am not sure how much importance should be attached to them.

I. H. Mills

It may be quite important to differentiate between adrenaline and noradrenaline. The main difference between exercise and mental stimulation is that exercise chiefly increases noradrenaline output, whereas mental stimulation chiefly puts up adrenaline output. Although we cannot explain all the effects, I believe that the stimulation of adrenaline output may be of much greater importance than that of noradrenaline. It may be very helpful to investigate this difference.

H. Keen

Are there different patterns of hormonal response for the same sort of psychic stimulus in different people? On one very stressful occasion—when I was taking the MRCP examination—I collected aliquots of urine over the 24 hours and the catecholamine content showed absolutely no elevation at all. On another occasion—when I was taking my MD—my cortisol and metabolite levels were about three times those found in the average case of Cushing's syndrome. Am I a cortical rather than a medullary reactor?

I. H. Mills

Yes, the pattern is very different not only in individuals under different circumstances, but in different individuals under the same circumstances. For instance, as regards your rise in cortisol production, the initial effect of stress is to increase the level of 5-hydroxytryptamine in the brain and stimulate ACTH release. But if the stress continues the 5-hydroxytryptamine slowly alters the "stat-point" in the brain, so ACTH production returns to normal. Stress does not raise steroid levels if it continues for months; then, as we have shown, the "stat-point" falls to an abnormally low level and steroid output may approach that seen in Addison's disease. When such individuals are treated with antidepressants for 4 months or so, the "stat-point" comes back up to normal again. Women who readily stop LH production when under stress, get amenorrhoea and may complain of infertility as a result. Women who are born with rather higher levels of LH production which are not readily stopped under stress may become hirsute; we have investigated all the biochemical pathways involved in that effect.

So there are indeed very big differences between individuals. In the case of prolactin there are even bigger differences. Some women release large quantities of prolactin day and night; they never ovulate, whereas others have short sharp rises in prolactin. Investigation of the different patterns may be of considerable importance in understanding the ultimate effects.

T. Theorell

I agree about the importance of the difference between adrenaline and noradrenaline output. One advantage of the measurement of urinary catecholamines is that it gives a relatively simple, integrated picture of arousal during a given period.

Cardiovascular Measures in Anxiety (Abstract)

D. R. MASTER

The Maudsley Hospital, London

The use of physiological techniques in the evaluation of psychiatric disorders has for many years appealed to researchers because of the possibility of establishing reliable diagnostic indices. However, the relationship between physiological measures and anxiety is still unclear, despite both the volume of research and the claims that there is an established relationship. The types of physiological measures studied may broadly be categorized as autonomic, somatic, and endocrine. In the work reported below, we have studied some of the autonomic measures in anxiety, particularly cardiovascular responses.

The most widely used measure has been heart rate. Less commonly, blood pressure and regional blood flow have been studied in anxious subjects. The usual experimental procedures in these studies are measurement of resting levels of the various indices, measurement of responses to various stimuli, both neutral and aversive, and measurement of the decrement in rate of response on repeated presentation of a stimulus.

An alternative approach to the study of physiological responses in subjects with trait anxiety is to investigate how response patterns become modified in anxiety states. This is most conveniently accomplished by the use of fear-evoking stimuli in phobic subjects. In such studies, differential heart-rate responses to various stimuli have been observed, with accelerative and decelerative components (Graham and Clifton, 1966). The accelerative response is generally held to be part of the self-explanatory defensive response or "startle" reaction, whilst the decelerative response is generally considered part of the orienting reflex, which accompanies attention to any stimulus not yet evaluated.

The hypothesis has been put by Sokolov (1963) that, if both neutral stimuli and anxiety-evoking stimuli are presented simultaneously, the orienting reflex can be inhibited by the defensive response. To test whether "background anxiety" affects the orienting reflex, at the Maudsley Hospital we have been studying a group of phobic subjects, mainly volunteers with specific animal phobias.

To elicit the orienting reflex we used a number of slides which had previously been shown to normal subjects who had considered their content pleasant and had responded by a deceleration in heart rate, indicating the orienting reflex. Our phobic subjects were then allocated at random to 3 groups:

1. a "no fear" group, to whom the "pleasant" slides mentioned above were presented for 10 s each without any concurrent phobic stimulus;
2. a "mild fear" group who, before being shown these "pleasant" slides, were exposed to a phobic stimulus at a distance sufficient to elicit what was rated as 50% fear; and
3. a "high fear" group who, before seeing the "pleasant" slides, were exposed to a phobic stimulus at a distance sufficient to elicit 100% fear, this being the maximum fear which the subject could tolerate.

The stimulus was applied in mid-expiration in half the subjects, and mid-expiration in the other half, and heart rate, skin conductance and respiratory activity measured while the slides were being shown. For purposes of comparison, control trials were first carried out before each of the experiments, the stimuli being applied at the

The Cardiovascular, Metabolic and Psychological Interface: Royal Society of Medicine International Congress and Symposium Series No. 14, published jointly by Academic Press Inc. (London) Ltd., and the Royal Society of Medicine.

same moment in the respective respiratory cycles and for the same length of time.

There were thus 6 sets of results, which were averaged; control results were subtracted from the subsequent experimental trial results, to give difference scores which reflected changes in heart rate unvitiated by effects due to sinus arrhythmia.

The results are at present being analysed, but it seems likely that under the conditions of the trial:

1. the "no fear" group will show deceleration of heart rate;
2. the "mild fear" group will show a deterioration in the deceleration response; and
3. the "high fear" group will show a greater deterioration in the deceleration response and perhaps even a frank defensive response.

References

Graham, F. K. and Clifton, R. K. (1966). Heart rate changes as a component of the orienting response. *Psychol. Bull.* **65**, 305–320.
Sokolov, E. N. (1963). Perception and the conditioned reflex. Pergamon Press, Oxford.

Discussion
I. H. Mills

Comparison of very short-term stimuli with real-life situations raises a problem: if one concentrates on the anxiety produced by short-lived stimuli one tends to think that the patient can be satisfactorily treated with anxiolytics such as the benzodiazepines. From the endocrinological point of view, the picture is entirely different. I see a large number of people with endocrine disturbance who have been treated with varying, sometimes very large doses of benzodiazepines and related drugs, and their endocrine status remains totally unaltered. I think we might change the concept: these episodes are really challenges to their coping mechanism, which I believe is related to different aspects of brain function, and when we give such patients tricyclic antidepressants, we find that not only does their endocrine status come back to normal but their actual coping is improved too; for instance, agoraphobics will go out and do their shopping normally. I think that we have to be careful when comparing short-term studies on anxiety with long-term effects which might be related to cardiovascular effects.

D. R. Master

I entirely agree. This sort of work really has no relevance to long-term anxiety and in a sense it is a slight departure from what has been dealt with previously. It is much more relevant to information processing. The currently held notions about information processing and heart rate are that attention to stimuli is facilitated by deceleration in heart rate, and rejection of stimuli is associated with acceleration of heart rate. This has much more to do with perceptual sensitivity and intake or rejection of stimuli than with anxiety as a clinical diagnosis.

M. Carruthers

I am very concerned about the use of heart rate as a psycho-physiological measure, because it is an end-stage of many conflicting factors. For example, while adrenaline speeds it up, noradrenaline may be reflexly slowing it down by raising blood pressure. In addition there is the vagal effect, which can be very large indeed; for example, during free-fall parachuting, one man landed with a heart rate of about 170 beats/min, but broke his ankle, and within a minute this had slowed down to 60 or 70 beats/min. When we showed subjects scenes of violence on film, we found they had high catecholamine levels but low heart rates. Similarly, highly aroused subjects sitting in a dentist's chair secreting large quantities of adrenaline in fact had slowing of the heart rate. So I think heart rate is a very complex measure which is difficult to interpret.

D. R. Master

Yes, I would accept most of what you said. I think the philosophical basis for looking at heart rate in this way has really stemmed from the Lacey concept of an association between cardiac activity and a tendency either to take in or reject stimuli. The so-called visual-afferent feedback theory has been proposed to account for phasic heart rate changes of this sort and this is derived from neurophysiological evidence that baroreceptor activities from the aortic arch and carotid sinuses have an inhibitory function on the cortex. However, I do realize that is an inadequate explanation of the criticisms you brought up.

Psychiatric Aspects of Hypertension (Abstract)

A. H. MANN

Institute of Psychiatry, London

The vascular changes noted as part of the physiological response to stress have stimulated interest in the potential role of psychological factors in the causation of hypertension for over 40 years. Investigations have followed two main lines: the relationship of psychiatric disorders or symptoms to the hypertensive state, and the identification of any personality type characteristic of that state.

The finding of Sainsbury (1960) that hypertensive outpatients at a hospital had more neurotic symptoms than other patients attending the medical outpatients department gave some impetus to the belief that an association existed between hypertension and minor psychiatric disorders. There have been many studies of such an association, but some have been handicapped by the fact that known hypertensive patients were interviewed. This made any finding open to the objection that being diagnosed hypertensive might be responsible for increased neurotic symptoms.

Forty years ago Alexander suggested that hypertensives tend to hide hostile feelings rather than express them, and that this tendency leads in time to permanently heightened vascular tone. This "repressed hostility" concept gained credence, receiving some support from laboratory experiments and uncontrolled clinical studies. But a major handicap in testing the concept has been the absence of a valid instrument for assessing hostility.

In the pilot phase of the MRC therapeutic trial for mild to moderate hypertension, a large number of subjects, both those found to be hypertensive and the normotensive completed a self-administered questionnaire designed to detect minor psychiatric disorder. I have personally interviewed some of them to establish a psychiatric diagnosis. Information has been gained from these assessments on both the relative prevalence of psychiatric symptoms in a hypertensive population and on hostility in relation to hypertension.

Approximately 13,000 subjects completed the screening questionnaire, the General Health Questionnaire (Goldberg, 1970), immediately *before* having their blood pressure measured for the purposes of the hypertension trial. The findings in these subsequently deemed hypertensive and normotensive subjects are given in Tables 1 and 2. No relationship was found between the level of blood pressure and the prevalence of neurotic symptoms in those subjects ignorant of their blood pressure.

Table 1
The relationship of General Health Questionnaire (GHQ) response to blood pressure level at screening of 12,683 subjects between 35 and 64 years of age

	Number	% scoring above the cut-off point on the GHQ	95% confidence interval
Diastolic blood pressure below 90 mmHg	M 5519	17·7	(16·7–18·7)
	F 4786	24·6	(23·4–25·8)
Diastolic blood pressure at 90 mmHg or above	M 1347	19·4	(18·3–20·5)
	F 1041	24·4	(21·8–27·0)

No significant differences.

The Cardiovascular, Metabolic and Psychological Interface: Royal Society of Medicine International Congress and Symposium Series No. 14, published jointly by Academic Press Inc. (London) Ltd., and the Royal Society of Medicine.

Table 2

A comparison of General Health Questionnaire (GHQ) responses, in subjects between 35 and 64, between those with temporary elevation of blood pressure and those deemed hypertensive after two estimations

	Number	% scoring above the cut-off point on the GHQ	95% confidence interval
Temporarily raised pressure	M 681	18·1	(15·2–20·9)
	F 489	23·7	(19·9–27·5)
Definitely elevated pressure	M 533	19·5	(16·1–22·9)
	F 447	23·7	(19·8–27·7)

No significant differences.

A number of hypertensive subjects in the trial and a similar number of normotensive controls were interviewed personally to assess severity of psychiatric symptoms and make a diagnosis. As part of the interview, the subjects also completed a hostility questionnaire that has been well validated for use in psychiatric practice, the "Hostility—Direction of Hostility Questionnaire" (Foulds, 1965).

Some relationships were shown between hostility and hypertension in that, as a group, the hypertensives were less self-critical than the normotensive subjects. When hypertensive and normotensive subjects without neurotic symptoms were compared, a greater tendency to display hostility was found among the hypertensive subjects.

These methods and results have been published fully elsewhere (Mann, 1977). In summary, it seems that there is no association between the hypertensive state *per se* and neurotic symptoms, and that any such increase found must be consequent upon diagnosis. Some relationship was shown between responses to a well-validated hostility questionnaire and level of blood pressure, but the relationship was the inverse of that predicted by the "repressed hostility" theory.

References

Alexander, F. (1939). Emotional factors in arterial hypertension. *Psychosom. Med.* **1**, 1973.

Foulds, G. (1965). "Personality and Personal Illness." Tavistock, London.

Goldberg, D. P. (1970). "Detection of Psychiatric Illnesses by Questionnaire." Maudsley Monograph. Oxford University Press, London.

Mann, A. H. (1977). Psychiatric morbidity and hostility in hypertension. *Psychol. Med.* **7**, 653–659.

Sainsbury, P. (1960). Neuroticism and hypertension in an outpatient population. *J. psychosom. Res.* **8**, 255.

Discussion

D. Ballantyne

Does the scoring on either of these questionnaires vary according to when it is answered?

A. H. Mann

For the general health questionnaire, the reliability is good. For the hostility questionnaire, re-test reliability obviously depends on again controlling for the subjects' psychiatric state. I do not know whether the individual rates himself in the same way on different occasions, but it has been shown that self-rating fluctuates with the level of depression.

T. Theorell

We have had the opportunity of examining Swedish 18-year-olds who undergo compulsory health screening for miltary service. One of the methods we used was to give them questionnaires describing hostility and inhibition of aggression. In these young people, despite small samples, we have observed significantly more inhibition of aggression in those with elevated blood pressure than in the normotensive. Might there be age differences relevant to hypertension?

A. H. Mann

I am not familiar with your hostility questionnaire: does the score relate to anxiety or to depression? The score on the Foulds questionnaire changes a great deal according to how anxious or depressed the subject is.

R. H. Rosenman

In a study of children in, I believe, Iowa, significant correlations between blood pressure levels and psychological factors such as aggression have been shown. The more aggressive they were, the higher their blood pressure.

H. Keen

We are very familiar with the fallacies which can result from the use of small numbers; may I utter a warning against the fallacies of using very large numbers? If enough observations are made, everything correlates significantly with everything else. With a million observations, it would be extraordinary if any two variates did not correlate significantly. Assessing the strength and the mechanism of the relationship is, of course, a very different matter. Secondly there is the difficulty the epidemiologists call "confounding variables". Suppose a relationship is found—or is not found—between mental state and blood pressure level (and both are related to age), could the interrelationship, or lack of it, between blood pressure and mental state be due to a confounding effect of age?

A. H. Mann

In the large-scale general health questionnaire study I looked at age in the various 5-year bands and found no relationship with blood pressure.

H. Keen

I should like to raise the question of separating data. If you take a list of observations, presumably unimodally distributed, and draw a line across the middle, and then say that those observations below a certain level indicate absence of disease and those above indicate presence of disease, you may be comparing subjects who are closely similar in respect of the variable in which you are interested. If you were to take patients at the extremes of the ranges of those distributions—those who on your scale were hypotensive, for example, and those at the upper end of the MRC category of moderate hypertension—might you then find a difference between psychological attributes? And what about heterogeneity? We talk about hypertension as if it were a single disease, which of course it is not; it is a syndrome or state arising from many precursor mechanisms. Could it be that within your major group you have a sub-set in which suppression of hostility is responsible for hypertension, and that this effect is diluted in the analysis by the large proportion of other hypertensives?

A. H. Mann

I suppose that may be so. As regards your previous point, I looked at the lower end of the MRC range (90–109 mmHg), comparing borderline cases with those at the upper end of the range and still there is no relationship to general health questionnaire scores. Whether or not there is a variant of personality which is associated with hypertension and is one aspect of people who repress hostility, I do not know. What I was really attacking was the use of this theory as a simplistic sociological explanation for people developing hypertension. There is very little evidence to justify that.

G. A. MacGregor

One of the problems of the MRC trial is that among the hypertensive subjects so designated after three measurements, who were then observed or treated with a placebo, there was a further fall in blood pressure so that after 6 months many of them became normotensive, as defined by your criteria. It would be much more profitable to study a group of more severely hypertensive patients to try and find correlations between levels of blood pressure and your indices, rather than cut-off points that do not exist.

A. H. Mann

Over a period of about 3–4 weeks after their first attendance patients would return to the clinic to have their blood pressure checked again; there were some whose blood pressure had settled meanwhile and these formed one group, while those whose diastolic pressure remained above 90 mmHg and within the trial range made up another. People who were known to be severely hypertensive were not included in the study but were referred for treatment without delay. The relationship of general health questionnaire score to blood pressure level in a person who is severely hypertensive is a different question altogether, and would require study of cerebral function to assess how far the mental state reflects cerebral damage (arteriopathy encephalopathy, and so on), when the blood pressure is very high.

G. A. MacGregor

Do I understand correctly that many of your hypertensive group became normotensive after a period of observation and that you have included them in your hypertensive group? Should they really be classified as hypertensive, do you think?

A. H. Mann

We did include them in the hypertensive group, but it is difficult to be certain whether they should be so classified. If a patient's blood pressure remains raised for 6 months, for example, and then goes down, would that mean he was hypertensive or not?

Metabolic Responses to Stress
(Abstract)

M. CARRUTHERS

The Maudsley Hospital, London

There is evidence that the acceleration of the normal deterioration with age of many cardiovascular functions is caused by excessive or unbalanced sympathetic activity, giving rise to a range of what could be termed "hypercatabolic diseases".

Patients with cardiovascular disease show evidence of increased sympathetic activity and decreased parasympathetic activity (Table 1). There is often evidence of a hyperkinetic circulation with raised pulse rate and blood pressure. This is usually associated with increased production, often stress-related, of hormones with a predominantly catabolic action such as catecholamines and corticosteroids. These have wide-ranging effects on lipid and carbohydrate metabolism, with repercussions through the cardiovascular system.

In the short term the most important change is mobilization of free fatty acids, which increase tissue oxygen consumption, promote the arrhythmogenic action of catecholamines and increase platelet adhesiveness. The long-term effects also contribute to atheroma formation by raising cholesterol and triglyceride levels (Fig. 1). These changes, and ways of modifying them, have been extensively studied in relation to theories linking emotion and cardiovascular disease. Less well documented are their effects on the subfractions of high-density lipoproteins.

Table 1
Autonomic factors in cardiovascular disease

	Sympathetic dominance	Parasympathetic dominance
Promoting factors	Stress (emotional, physical, thermal) Surgery Smoking	Physical training Mental training (Autogenic training and yoga) Sleep
Metabolic effects	Catabolic	Anabolic
Testosterone and insulin	Decreased	Increased
Fibrinolytic activity	Decreased	Increased
Catecholamines and corticosteroids	Increased	Decreased
Lipids, glucose and uric acid	Increased	Decreased
Heart rate and blood pressure	Increased	Decreased
Signs and symptoms of tissue hypoxia (e.g. angina, limb pain, ST–T depression)	Increased	Decreased

The Cardiovascular, Metabolic and Psychological Interface: Royal Society of Medicine International Congress and Symposium Series No. 14, published jointly by Academic Press Inc. (London) Ltd., and the Royal Society of Medicine.

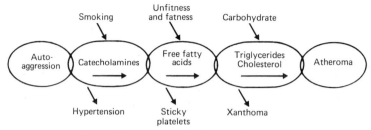

Figure 1. Factors contributing to atherogenesis.

These patients also show signs of a decrease in parasympathetic activity and corresponding reduction in hormones with mainly anabolic effects, particularly testosterone and insulin. Male patients with early atherosclerosis have been found to have reduced testosterone production, as have subjects with overt coronary disease. The latter also have high oestradiol levels. As well as physical trauma, a variety of different forms of emotional stress, including even aircraft noise, have been shown to reduce testosterone production.

Contrary to what was expected from the low incidence of coronary disease in pre-menopausal women, administration of oestrogens to either sex can predispose to venous or arterial thrombosis. Oestradiol itself can cause depression of the ST segment on the electrocardiogram.

Anabolic steroids given to patients with advanced circulatory disease, which can be regarded as replacement therapy, can have a "parasympathetic" action which reverses many of the associated physiological and biochemical changes. The patients show reduced pulse rates and blood pressure, though this may also be contributed to by the increased physical activity which is encouraged. As well as there being a decrease in symptoms and signs of tissue hypoxia, fibrinolytic activity and carbohydrate tolerance are increased. Insulin requirements in diabetes fall, and non-diabetics may also experience hypoglycaemic episodes.

Sympathetic predominance is seen in its most severe and acute form following major surgery. There is intense catabolic activity with a negative nitrogen balance and increased ACTH, catecholamine and corticosteroid production, which often continues for 1–2 weeks after surgery. During this period there is also evidence of decreased parasympathetic activity, with a lowering of testosterone and insulin levels, and impaired glucose tolerance and fibrinolytic activity. These changes are remarkably similar to those seen in cardiovascular disease, and so it is not surprising that arterial and venous thromboses are some of the most common complications in the post-operative period.

Discussion
G. E. Foster

At what age does lowering the blood cholesterol, by whatever means, help to spare the coronary arteries? Are those of us who are in our thirties and faithfully eat polyunsaturated margarine closing the stable door long after the horse has bolted.

M. Carruthers

Yes, I think it may already be too late. I have looked for, but not found, practical evidence that limiting one's major pleasures in life, in which I would include diet, can produce a worthwhile improvement in coronary risk.

D. Ballantyne

I gather you were suggesting that there is no relationship between diet and plasma cholesterol levels, and you quoted Mann as stating this opinion recently. Mann has published articles along these lines and my own view is that he has misinterpreted his data. In a recent review Stamler, using the same evidence, comes to the entirely opposite conclusion that there is a relationship between diet and coronary heart disease and cholesterol, and therefore between cholesterol and coronary heart disease.

Now, as regards the evidence that it does any good to change the cholesterol levels, there are two relevant studies that I know of: the Veterans Administration

Study carried out in Los Angeles, and the mental hospital study in Finland. Both can be criticized but both showed that changing the diet did indeed reduce the risk of coronary heart disease.

If I could just make one other point: Fig. 1 shows the chain of events leading to atheroma and an arrow leading from "triglycerides and cholesterol" to "xanthoma". I can accept that aggression or auto-aggression can cause change in the cholesterol and triglyceride levels but I cannot accept that this can cause xanthoma, because these lesions are only found in very severely hypercholesterolaemic patients and always have a genetic basis. So I cannot accept that emotion can cause xanthoma.

M. Carruthers

Perhaps I was using the word xanthoma too loosely to imply lipid deposition in the tissues in general, rather than just in the skin or around the eyes. It would take far too long for us to discuss all the evidence for and against the dietary hypothesis here, but the more closely one looks at the balance of all the evidence, the less likely does it seem that there is a simple dietetic relationship. As I pointed out earlier, there is a good correlation between fat intakes in various countries and the heart disease rates obtaining in those countries. I was trying to emphasize what I believe to be indirect associations; for example, one can also plot heart attack rates against number of television licences or against number of motor vehicle licences, and find fairly close correlations here as well. The more one looks at the dietetic studies that have been reported, the more imperfect and inconclusive they seem, and the theory that coronary heart disease is a direct consequence of dietary factors seems to be losing popularity among its former adherents.

R. J. Jarrett

We have had two presentations which have selected epidemiological evidence to support their case. Speaking as an epidemiologist relatively uncommitted in this particular field, I would point out the enormous complexity of epidemiological associations in relation to coronary heart disease. First of all there is the actual diagnostic problem in coronary heart disease; secondly, there is the fact that associations are different with different aspects of coronary heart disease. With angina, or sudden death, or myocardial infarction with or without survival, the epidemiological associations are different. One also has the problem that within populations there are very different specific mortalities in different occupations. Even within medicine, for instance, there are quite large differences between the coronary heart disease mortality rates of general practitioners and surgeons, general practitioners having the higher rate, and surgeons quite a low one. Of course, there are also big differences within the profession in deaths from other causes, such as suicide. I hate to say this in present company, but I believe psychiatrists have the highest mortality from suicide.

These differences in specific mortality are in part due to environmental factors in the occupation itself, and in part to the type of personality of the individual selecting the particular occupation. To that extent I would not deny that personality traits are likely to be associated with the risk of coronary heart disease but I would submit that they only explain some of the variations in already high coronary heart disease rates. Dr Carruthers played down the role of cholesterol here. Now there is no doubt that cholesterol levels do not explain all the variations we see in coronary heart disease rates, but one cannot get away from the fact that those populations in which coronary heart disease is very infrequent are populations with low cholesterol levels. Dr Carruthers was referring to levels of 180, 190 and 200 mg/100 ml as being normal or low; they are not normal or low, they are high. Levels in relatively undeveloped countries are 130 mg/100 ml or lower, the maximum being 130; in the study which I quoted yesterday of the vegetarians in Boston, average levels were 130 mg/100 ml. That is what I would regard as normal. Anything above that is high, and the vast majority of people with episodes of coronary heart disease are going to come from among those with what we call normal levels of cholesterol, that is, in the range of 170 to 230 mg/100 ml, because that is what most people have. Levels of 250 mg/100 ml or above make up the top 10% or thereabouts of cholesterol levels and they are not just high, they are *very* high.

M. Carruthers

Again, I was trying to point out the differences between associations and between truly causal factors, and to illustrate one in relation to cholesterol, and the other in relation to free fatty acids. I think we must again emphasize the difference between dietary cholesterol and levels of circulating plasma cholesterol. They are almost talked of in the same breath, but there is a vast difference between them, for only 20–25% of plasma cholesterol comes directly from the diet.

Lipoproteins and Coronary Heart Disease (Abstract)

B. I. HOFFBRAND

Whittington Hospital, London

The belief that plasma cholesterol plays a major role in the development of coronary heart disease (CHD) comes from a wealth of pathological, epidemiological, clinical and experimental observations, some dating from the nineteenth century. Advances in laboratory methods led to definition of the lipoprotein fractions carrying cholesterol and other blood lipids around 1950 (Fig. 1). Low-density lipoprotein (LDL) carries the bulk (normally about 70%) of circulating

Electrophoretic separation	α	β	pre-β	Chylomicron
Density	HDL (high density lipoprotein)	LDL (low density lipoprotein)	VLDL (very low density lipoprotein)	chylomicron
Size		S small	M medium	L large
Average composition	45% 26% 8% 21%	21% 18% 51% 10%	7% 21% 18% 54%	4% 1% 9% 86%

Protein □ Phospholipid ■ Triglyceride ▨ Cholesterol ▤

Figure 1. Features of the phospholipid fractions.

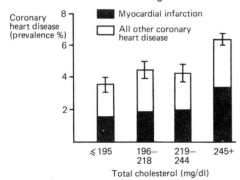

Coronary heart disease (prevalence %)

■ Myocardial infarction
□ All other coronary heart disease

Total cholesterol (mg/dl): ≤195, 196–218, 219–244, 245+

Figure 2. Relationship of coronary heart disease to total cholesterol levels (from Rhoads et al., 1976).

cholesterol and shows the same relationships as plasma total cholesterol to CHD (Fig. 2). Very-low-density lipoprotein (VLDL) carries roughly 13% of the plasma cholesterol and is probably no more closely related to CHD than might be expected from its cholesterol content. VLDL carries the bulk of the plasma triglycerides in the fasting state but the relationship of plasma triglyceride levels to CHD is uncertain and probably not of major importance.

Recently, interest has centred on high-density lipoprotein (HDL) carrying roughly 17% or so of the plasma total cholesterol. Numerous observations since the first days of lipoprotein analysis have shown an *inverse* relationship between

The Cardiovascular, Metabolic and Psychological Interface: Royal Society of Medicine International Congress and Symposium Series No. 14, published jointly by Academic Press Inc. (London) Ltd., and the Royal Society of Medicine.

HDL, measured as either its cholesterol or protein fractions, and CHD. However, widespread interest in HDL was not aroused until the paper of Miller and Miller (1975), who stressed the association between CHD and low HDL levels and reviewed the evidence that many of the risk factors for CHD are associated with reduced HDL concentrations. They also reported that body cholesterol pools were negatively correlated with plasma HDL concentration but unrelated to plasma cholesterol and levels of the other lipoproteins.

In addition to considerable case-control data on the association of CHD with low HDL levels, there is evidence that apparently well individuals with low HDL levels are more likely to develop CHD than controls with higher levels. HDL cholesterol is now believed to be more valuable than LDL cholesterol in predicting CHD. The two variables are more or less independent and prognostic indices incorporating both measurements have been devised, although the value of such indices in practice has yet to be assessed. The hypothesis that HDL cholesterol is protective is reinforced by observations of families with considerably elevated HDL levels and a prevalence of CHD significantly lower than expected. There is experimental evidence which suggests mechanisms by which HDL could be anti-atherogenic, by increasing uptake of cholesterol from peripheral tissues for catabolism and excretion by the liver, and by inhibiting tissue uptake of cholesterol-rich LDL.

HDL levels show no consistent change with age but are higher in women than men. This difference may be hormonal, as oestrogens raise and androgens lower plasma HDL concentrations.

Changes in lipoprotein concentrations in subjects taking oral contraceptives depend on the composition of the particular preparation. HDL concentrations rise with physical activity (Table 1)

Table 1
The effect of exercise on blood lipid levels (mg/100ml) (from Wood et al., 1974).

	Runners	Controls
Total cholesterol	200	210
Triglycerides	70	146
HDL cholesterol	64	43
LDL cholesterol	125	139
Ratio $\dfrac{\text{HDL cholesterol}}{\text{LDL cholesterol}}$	0·51	0·31

and with alcohol consumption, but are reduced in hypercholesterolaemias, obesity and untreated insulin-deficient diabetics. The complex metabolic interrelations between HDL on the one hand and VLDL and triglyceride metabolism on the other may be relevant to these and other observations concerning plasma HDL concentrations.

Although there is evidence that HDL may be an important mechanism by means of which a number of risk factors for CHD operate, differences in HDL concentrations are not related to hypertension and smoking, and cannot explain differences in prevalence of CHD between certain ethnic groups. The crucial experiment of raising plasma HDL concentrations and reducing the prevalence of CHD has yet to be performed. This would require a nontoxic means of increasing HDL production by the liver. Current drugs have little to offer in this respect.

References

Castelli, W. P., Doyle, J. T., Gordon, T., Hames, C. G., Hjortland, M. C., Halley, S. B., Kagan, A. and Zukel, W. J. (1977). HDL cholesterol and other lipids in coronary heart disease. The co-operative lipoprotein phenotyping study. *Circulation* **55**, 767–772.

Davignon, J. (1978). The lipid hypothesis. Pathophysiological basis. *Arch. Surg.* **113**, 29–34

Miller, G. J. and Miller, N. E. (1975). Plasma high density lipoprotein concentration and development of ischaemic heart disease. *Lancet* **1**. 16–19.

Rhoads, G. G., Gullbrandsen, C. L. and Kagan, A. (1976). Serum lipoproteins and coronary heart disease in a population study of Hawaii Japanese men. *New Engl. J. Med.* **294**, 293–298.

Wood, D. D., Klein, H., Lewis, S. and Haskell, W. L. (1974). Plasma lipoprotein concentrations in middle-aged male runners. Abstracts of 47th Scientific Sessions of the American Heart Association. *Circulation* **50** (Suppl. 3). Abstract No. 452, p. 115.

Discussion
R. J. Jarrett

You did not mention diet, which I think is important, as it also brings up the relationship between HDL cholesterol and total cholesterol. This has been studied in vegetarians, in whom the HDL cholesterols were found to be lower than in a control population eating an ordinary mixed Western-type diet. Of course the LDL cholesterols were very much lower. The actual ratio was different, which brings up one of the points in the Framingham work, which suggests that it is the ratio of HDL to LDL cholesterol that is important, rather than the absolute levels.

B. I. Hoffbrand

I agree. I deliberately did not go into the dietary aspects; bran apparently does not raise HDL cholesterol levels. The point you make about a vegetarian diet probably being beneficial is very important.

P. G. F. Nixon

I agree with Professor Mills that health can be described by curves representing phases of high arousal and deteriorating performance, as shown in Fig. 1 associated with gross and bizarre disturbances of the internal milieu. Huge disturbances of the lipids and the blood pressure take place during the phase represented by the downward slope. Now if these disturbances are important risk factors, it follows logically that behaviour is a very important risk factor, for a man is free to choose whether to live on the downward slope or on the upward slope. No study of lipids and blood

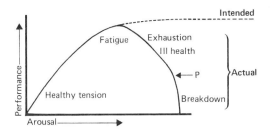

Figure 1. Scheme of the human function curve. P = The point at which even minimal arousal may precipitate a breakdown.

pressure published so far indicates where the individual cases are on that curve—whether in high or low arousal—and therefore the results are quite impossible to interpret as far as individual patients are concerned.

D. Ballantyne

May I come back to the question of diet and HDL? I think it is true that if a subject has abnormal lipids to start with, the HDL level can be altered fairly easily, particularly if the triglyceride level is high, but if one tries to treat a whole population of people with normal lipids, it is very difficult to raise the HDL level; I think this limits the usefulness of the low HDL cholesterol level as a risk factor. In normal people with normal lipids, it is difficult to do anything about it.

B. I. Hoffbrand

But it is very difficult to be sure what we really mean by normal. It is probable that we have all got high blood total cholesterol levels and that the 5 % at the upper end of the scale is really only the tip of the iceberg of increased risk.

Beta-blockade and Diabetes Mellitus
(Extended Abstract)

H. KEEN, G. C. VIBERTI and R. SALGADO

Unit for Metabolic Medicine,
Guy's Hospital, London

It has been suggested that beta-adrenergic blockade may mask the warning symptoms of hypoglycaemia, increase its severity or delay recovery, and so may be contraindicated in diabetics, especially the insulin-treated. It may also interfere with glycogenolysis, pancreatic release of glucagon or insulin, levels of circulating free fatty acids and perhaps peripheral metabolism, and act on other hormone or substrate concentrations involved in glucose metabolism in the diabetic (Day, 1975). These views have been based on evidence from case reports (Feely, 1977) or observations (e.g. Davidson et al., 1977) in non-diabetics, however, and the effects of beta-blockade on diabetics have seldom been studied directly under controlled conditions. We have therefore investigated the effects of beta-blockade on glucose metabolism in normal subjects and diabetics in two sets of experiments and this is a preliminary report of our findings.

First Study

To compare the effect of beta-blockade by oxprenolol on disposal of an oral glucose load with that of placebo, four groups of patients were investigated:

Group 1. 11 non-diabetic controls (aged 21–44),
Group 2. 7 diabetics (aged 43–76) treated by diet alone,
Group 3. 12 diabetics (aged 27–71) receiving oral anti-diabetic agents, and
Group 4. 11 diabetics (aged 21–67) treated with insulin.

Subjects were given either placebo or oxprenolol 40 mg 8-hourly for 6 doses, the final dose being taken on the morning of the test after an overnight fast. Group 3 subjects took their usual medication and the test drug 1 h before the 50 g glucose load. Group 4 subjects took the test drug 1 h before and their insulin 15 min before the glucose load.

Blood was taken at intervals for determination of sugar, insulin, free fatty acid and growth hormone levels, and the adequacy of beta-blockade assessed by inhibition of acceleration of pulse rate induced by glyceryl trinitrate 0·5 mg sublingually.

In all groups blood sugar levels were slightly but not significantly higher with blockade than without (Fig. 1); they were accompanied by, and were probably due to, the lowered insulin values observed (Fig. 2) in the normal subjects, particularly in the initial response.

Baseline plasma non-esterified fatty acid (NEFA) levels did not differ significantly according to treatment with active or inert agent (Fig. 3), but after the glucose load they remained somewhat higher with beta-blockade, probably owing to diminution of insulin release and its anti-lipolytic effect. In insulin-dependent subjects, in whom similar trends were observed with oxprenolol, other factors such as agonist action, peripheral metabolic effects or even residual insulin secretion were probably also involved.

Second Study

To investigate the effects of oxprenolol and metoprolol on induction of and recovery from insulin-

The Cardiovascular, Metabolic and Psychological Interface: Royal Society of Medicine International Congress and Symposium Series No. 14, published jointly by Academic Press Inc. (London) Ltd., and the Royal Society of Medicine.

34

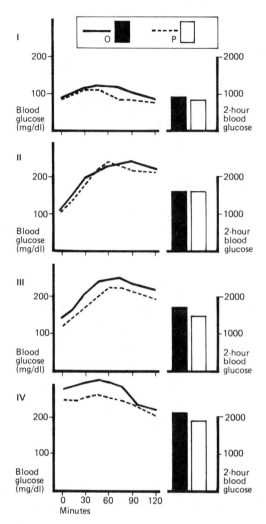

Figure 1. Glycaemic response to 50 g oral glucose load in normal controls (I), diet-treated diabetics (II), oral-agent-treated diabetics (III) and insulin-treated diabetics (IV). Blood glucose concentration (mg/dl) shown on vertical scale at left of each panel and 2-h blood glucose area in arbitrary units (mg/dl × time) at right of each panel. Time (min) on abscissa. Open symbols denote blood glucose values after placebo (P) and solid symbols after oxprenolol (O). Columns at right of each panel show area under curve of blood sugar.

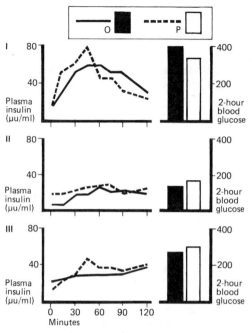

Figure 2. Insulinaemic response corresponding to glucose response in Fig. 1. Insulin in μu/ml on left-hand vertical axis, insulinaemic area under curve on right-hand vertical axis in arbitrary units (μu/ml × time). Estimations were not carried out for insulin-treated patients. Symbols for placebo and oxprenolol treatments as for Fig. 1.

Following an overnight fast, insulin was infused i.v. with a priming dose of 3 u followed by 6 u/h, blood glucose being monitored at frequent intervals. The infusion was stopped when symptoms of hypoglycaemia arose or the blood glucose level fell below 36 mg/100 ml; in diabetics this took much longer than in controls (about 120 min as against 30 min) owing to higher initial levels in the diabetics. NEFA, growth hormone and catecholamine levels were measured throughout the infusion and for 1–2 h after. Pulse rate, blood pressure, degree of sweating, and other effects were also recorded.

Response of blood glucose

Blood glucose concentration fell steadily with infusion in both controls and diabetics (2·25 and 2·33 mg/100 ml/min respectively), but in diabetics, as it entered the range of normal (from 80 mg/100 ml down), the rate of fall slowed to 0·9 mg/100 ml/min. Over this range the rate of fall was slightly slower in controls and diabetics taking oxprenolol

induced hypoglycaemia, eight normal subjects and seven insulin-dependent diabetics (of 4–15 years' standing and without obvious ocular, renal, neurological or arterial complications) were subjected three times to insulin infusion as follows: 60 min after administration (in random order) of oxprenolol 80 mg, metoprolol 100 mg or placebo.

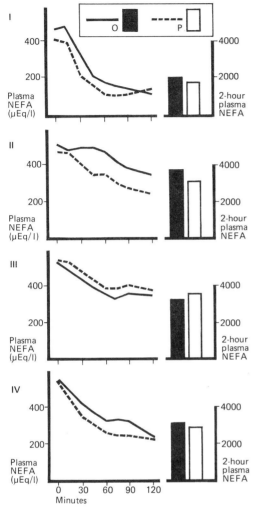

Figure 3. Non-esterified fatty acid (NEFA) response to glucose load corresponding to Figs 1 and 2 with the same symbol convention. Values on left-hand vertical axis in μEq/litre. Values denoting NEFA "areas" on right-hand axis in arbitrary units of mmol/litre × time.

and metoprolol than with those given placebo (Figs 4a and 4b).

After infusion, blood glucose levels in controls rose though the upturn in the curve occurred a few minutes later with beta-blockers than with placebo and values remained about 5 mg/100 ml lower throughout the recovery period. After infusion in the diabetics, however, blood sugar levels recovered very sluggishly, mean concentrations remaining below 40 mg/100 ml 1 h after it was stopped; blocking agents did not affect this rate of recovery.

Response of free fatty acids

NEFA levels fell with insulin infusion in controls and the rate of fall was unaffected by beta-blockade (Fig. 5a). When the infusion was discontinued, in the absence of blockade there was a prompt rise with some overshoot. However, with both blocking agents NEFA continued to fall (for about 40 min with oxprenolol and 20 min with metoprolol) before returning to normal levels. The subsequent rise took place in oxprenolol-treated subjects at a nearly normal rate but was slower in the metoprolol-treated. In diabetics, in whom initial NEFA levels were higher, insulin infusion provoked a fall in these levels which was unaffected by blockade but took place at only half the rate of that in controls (Fig. 5b). In the placebo-takers, after the infusion NEFA levels promptly rose (without overshoot) but in those given either beta-blocker the rise was clearly delayed.

Cardiovascular responses

In placebo-treated controls, 20 min of insulin infusion raised heart rate by 13 beats/min or more, but 20 min after infusion was discontinued it had returned to its base line value. Systolic pressure rose by about 8 mmHg, returning to its baseline value 30 min after; diastolic pressure was unchanged during infusion but fell slightly for 30 min after.

In beta-blocked controls, both agents abolished the infusion-induced tachycardia and caused systolic pressure to fall slightly during infusion and rise by 10 mmHg for about 30 min after; diastolic pressure behaved similarly with oxprenolol but with metoprolol there was no change in diastolic pressure.

By contrast, in placebo-treated diabetics there was little if any change in blood pressure or pulse rate with insulin. In those given either of the beta-blockers, systolic pressure slowly sank by 10 mmHg during infusion and picked up again by 30 min after it was stopped, and in none of these cases did hypoglycaemia provoke a rise in pressure.

Sweating

Neither beta-blocker greatly affected hypoglycaemia-induced sweating either in controls or diabetics; if anything, sweating was rather more prolonged in beta-blockade. Neither drug affected subjective responses to hypoglycaemia.

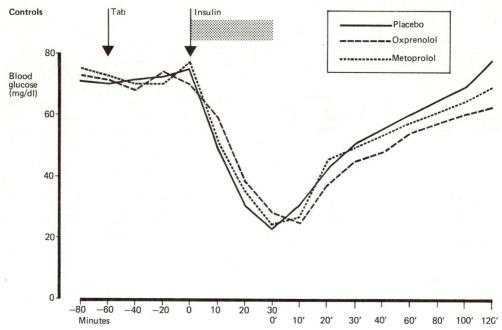

Figure 4a. Comparison of blood glucose concentration during and after intravenous insulin infusion in normal controls pretreated in random order with placebo, oxprenolol and metoprolol.

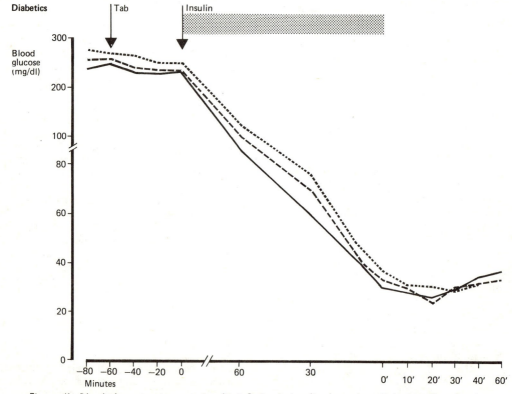

Figure 4b. Blood glucose response to insulin infusion in insulin-dependent diabetics after placebo, oxprenolol or metoprolol. The post-infusion hypoglycaemia was terminated after 1 h with oral glucose followed by food.

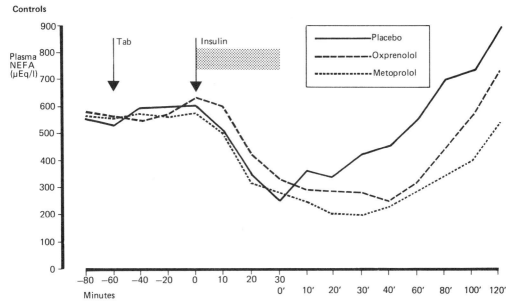

Figure 5a. The effect in normal controls of beta-blockade with oxprenolol or metoprolol compared with placebo on the response of plasma NEFA to insulin infusion and hypoglycaemia (same experiments as those illustrated in Fig. 4a).

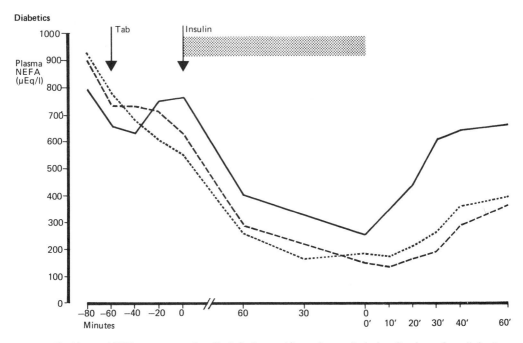

Figure 5b. Plasma NEFA response to insulin infusion and hypoglycaemia in insulin-dependent diabetics after treatment with placebo, oxprenolol or metoprolol (same experiments as those illustrated in Fig. 4b).

Discussion

These studies set out to answer two questions.

First: does beta-blockade, by blunting insulin release, provoke significant glucose intolerance? In other words, is it diabetogenic, or does it worsen existing diabetes where insulin secretion is compromised but not absent? Here, only trivial elevation of blood glucose levels were produced by oxprenolol.

Second (and more serious): do beta-blockers promote hypoglycaemia in diabetics, particularly in the insulin-dependent variety? The immediate counter-regulatory response to hypoglycaemia in man is largely glucagon-dependent, and this and the subsequent hepatic glycogenolysis is not influenced by cardioselective beta-blockers; catecholamine-induced glycogenolysis is probably mediated in man by alpha-adrenoceptors and is little affected by beta-blockade. Our findings highlighted the grossly defective counter-regulatory blood glucose response to hypoglycaemia in many established insulin-dependent diabetics regardless of beta-blockade.

The sweating response was intact and perhaps enhanced by beta-blockade.

It is not possible to extrapolate these findings to diabetics with brisk and intact counter-regulatory responses, and further investigations with more reactive patients are called for. Results may vary according to the beta-blocker used, length of treatment before study, and the presence of autonomic neuropathy. The dose of beta-blockers producing comparable degrees of blockade may be difficult to find, and there is a danger of insulin-induced hypertensive episodes in hypoglycaemic diabetics under beta-blockade, although this was not observed in the experiments reported above, while there may also be a risk to some diabetics of peripheral ischaemia from beta-blockade.

Until more is known about such hazards, it does in theory at least make sense to use beta-specific antagonists in insulin-dependent diabetics.

Conclusions

1. Non-selective beta-blockers produce mild but clinically insignificant impairment of glucose tolerance in normal subjects and diabetics.

2. This is probably due to some blunting of insulin release which also accounts for the slower FFA fall in blocked subjects after glucose.

3. Peripheral effects of beta-blocking agents and intrinsic sympathomimetic action may also play a role.

4. There is little acceptable published evidence of an increased risk of hypoglycaemia in insulin-dependent diabetics. In experimental studies, in normal subjects and insulin-dependent diabetics, the rate of glucose fall and the nadir achived were not affected either by oxprenolol or metoprolol compared with placebo. Blood glucose restoration in the diabetics was grossly defective both without and with beta-blockade.

5. Hypoglycaemia with beta-blockade is perhaps most likely to occur in the glycogen-depleted individual who depends on circulating gluconeogenic precursors, mainly from muscle, to maintain normal blood sugar levels.

Acknowledgement

We acknowledge the research support provided for these studies by Ciba Laboratories and our gratitude to the control and diabetic subjects involved. Requests for reprints of this abstract of the original paper should be addressed to H.K., Unit for Metabolic Medicine, Guy's Hospital, London SE1 9RT.

References

Davidson, N. McD., Corrall, R. J. M., Shaw, T. R. D. and French, E. B. (1977). Observations in man of hypoglycaemia during selective and non-selective beta-blockade. *Scot. med. J.* **22**, 69–72.

Day, J. L. (1975). The metabolic consequences of adrenergic blockade: a review. *Metabolism* **24**, 987–996.

Feely, J. (1977). Beta-blockers for diabetics. *Lancet* **2**, 950.

Discussion
K. Shaw

A practical problem I have encountered in treating insulin-dependent diabetics with beta-blockers is that the warning features of hypoglycaemia, on which many diabetics depend, may be abolished—so that they crash out without warning. I was therefore interested that the sweating response was preserved in your study of insulin-induced hypoglycaemia. Did your patients on beta-blockers develop symptoms of hypoglycaemia? And is there any difference between the types of beta-blockers which you studied?

H. Keen

Well, some diabetics crash out anyway, on beta-blockers or not, and it is difficult to say whether those on beta-blockers do so more frequently. So far as our studies were concerned, blockade seemed to make no difference to the subjective—mental or emotional—symptoms of hypoglycaemia. One thing that they did abolish was the pumping sensation from the heart, as I know from personal experience as one of the controls. Otherwise, beta-blockade made no difference to the sensations that accompanied hypoglycaemia, apart from the slight *increase* in sweating.

P. S. Sever

It is not surprising that the beta-blocking drugs have no effect on sweating because most sweat glands, although sympathetically innervated, are stimulated by acetyl-choline—on which beta-blockade would have no effect.

D. Leslie

At Kings we have done a prospective study on 33 insulin-dependent diabetics who were followed up for a mean period of two months; 32 of them experienced a total of 118 hypoglycaemic episodes, all with warning symptoms. On five occasions the patient actually blacked out, but on the other 113 occasions there was no loss of consciousness. Only one patient actually experienced loss of symptoms—including sweating—when taking a beta-blocker; that patient was on propranolol and re-gained warning symptoms when changed to metoprolol. Although these are pre-liminary results, the hesitation of physicians to put insulin-dependent diabetics on beta-blockers because of loss of warning symptoms appears to be misplaced.

N. Oakley

In connection with the delayed rise in blood glucose in the diabetic patients, there would of course have been more insulin infused than in the normals. Had these patients got high levels of insulin-binding antibodies? Had they been treated with highly purified insulins, and were you using highly purified pork insulins for your tests?

H. Keen

We certainly used mono-component porcine insulin for the tests, but most of those patients had been on ordinary insulin previously and were probably binding a good deal within the circulation. That may have accounted in part for the prolongation of hypoglycaemia. However, it was interesting to note that the insulin effect was not enough to stop patients not receiving a beta-blocker from getting quite a sharp rise in free fatty acid concentration.

Lipid Changes and Beta-blockade
(Abstract)

C. W. H. HAVARD

Royal Northern Hospital, London

Beta-adrenoreceptor antagonists inhibit catecholamine-induced lipolysis in adipose tissue and prevent the rise in plasma non-esterified fatty acids (NEFA). All beta-blockers antagonize the isoprenaline-induced increase in NEFA but the non-selective beta-blockers do so rather more effectively. In patients with myocardial infarction, plasma NEFA concentrations are higher in those who develop ventricular fibrillation, suggesting a possible arrhythmia-promoting effect of elevated NEFA concentrations in the blood. Triglyceride concentrations also appear to be important, as there is evidence that raised triglyceride concentrations increase the risk of cardiovascular death when they exceed 1·7 mmol/litre, irrespective of the cholesterol concentration. Raised NEFA and triglyceride levels may therefore be potentially harmful in hypertensive patients who are already at risk of cardiovascular disease.

There is currently much debate about whether beta-blockers or diuretics should be used as first-line treatment for moderate hypertension. They are both effective for lowering blood pressure, and it may be that the choice will depend on the adverse effects of prolonged treatment. The incidence of carbohydrate intolerance after diuretic therapy is significant, and diuretics may be associated with a rise in serum cholesterol concentrations. The effect of prolonged treatment with beta-blockers on lipid metabolism is therefore of importance.

Metoprolol Study

We have studied the effects of metoprolol 100 mg twice daily on fasting plasma lipids over a period of 12 weeks, in 15 selected outpatients with uncomplicated essential hypertension. The study was of single-blind design with 3 treatment periods preceded by a run-in period of 4 weeks in which no medication was given. In the first treatment period, a placebo was given for 4 weeks. In the second treatment period, metoprolol 100 mg twice daily was given for a period of 12 weeks. In the third and final period placebo was again given for 4 weeks. The placebo and active drug were identical in appearance and the times of administration were the same. Patients were seen at 2-weekly intervals and blood pressure was measured with a Hawksley random-zero sphygmomanometer. On the evening before attending the clinic, the patients were asked not to smoke or consume any alcohol and to take nothing but water after 22·00.

Twelve patients completed the study, and the main findings are shown in Table 1 and Fig. 1. The mean blood pressure and pulse rate at the end of the first placebo period were 156/104 mmHg and 74/min respectivley. At the end of metoprolol treatment these values fell to 127/83 mmHg and 60 beats/min. The mean triglyceride concentration was unchanged at 1·3 mmol/litre in each of the three treatment periods. The mean plasma NEFA concentration fell significantly 2 weeks after metoprolol was introduced and this fall remained consistent throughout the entire treatment period of 12 weeks. Two weeks after stopping metoprolol, the levels rose to pretreatment values. The NEFA concentration on placebo was 780 mmol/litre and on metoprolol 603 mmol/litre. Cholesterol levels were slightly increased on metoprolol treatment but this did not reach statistical significance. There was a slight but significant fall in serum

The Cardiovascular, Metabolic and Psychological Interface: Royal Society of Medicine International Congress and Symposium Series No. 14, published jointly by Academic Press Inc. (London) Ltd., and the Royal Society of Medicine.

Table 1
Main findings of metoprolol study

Day	28	118	140
Treatment	Placebo	Metoptolol	Placebo
BP	159/104	127[a]/83[a]	149/99
Pulse	75	60[b]	70
NEFA (mmol/litre)	760	553[b]	788
Cholesterol (mmol/litre)	5·8	6·3	5·9
Triglycerides (mmol/litre)	1·3	1·3	1·3
Albumin (g/litre)	41	38[a]	42
Globulin (g/litre)	23	24	22

[a] $P < 0.5$.   [b] $P < 0.01$.

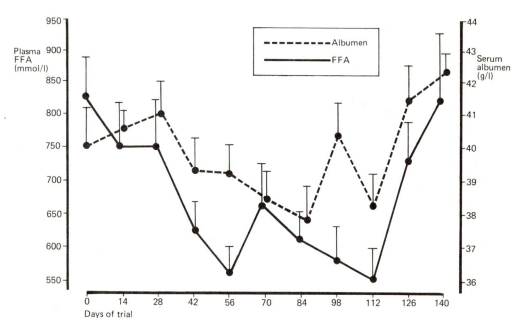

Figure 1. Effect of metoprolol on plasma free fatty acid and serum albumin levels in 15 patients with uncomplicated hypertension.

albumin concentration from 40·5 to 39·1 g/litre but the serum globulin concentration was unchanged by metoprolol. Body weight was unchanged.

Conclusions

Metoprolol, in doses which significantly reduce raised arterial blood pressure, has no effect on plasma triglyceride or cholesterol concentration but causes a significant reduction in plasma NEFA. This may be of advantage in patients with risk factors for myocardial infarction including those who are hypertensive. Metoprolol caused a small but significant fall in the serum albumin concentration. This is unlikely to be due to a dilution effect as the serum globulin concentration was unchanged. NEFA are avidly bound to albumin but the relationship is a stoichiometric one. The reduction in serum albumin (7%) would therefore not account for the much larger (27%) reduction in NEFA.

Discussion
M. Carruthers

Most of the studies done in high-adrenaline, high-anxiety situations do not appear to show an increase in free fatty acids—in contrast to more aggression-related situations the predominant amine is noradrenaline, which does appear to produce a rise in free fatty acids. I do not see how that fits in with my rather confused impression of what you said about $beta_1$ and $beta_2$ receptors and their specificity for these two catecholamines.

Secondly, I wonder how much the changes in albumin levels, for example, may be related to differences in physical activity? The normal plasma protein ranges for in-patients and outpatients are known to be different. Similarly, marginal hypercholesteraemia in a patient who comes in hot and steaming off the streets can be brought down into the normal range within 20 min simply by lying the patient down. The haemodilution of assuming the supine position promptly reduces the blood cholesterol level by 10 to 15%.

C. W. H. Havard

I cannot say how the specificity of $beta_1$ and $beta_2$ receptors relates to raised adrenaline and/or noradrenaline blood levels; we also need to ask what part alpha-receptors play. With regard to the possible effect of activity, there was no apparent change in activity during the study—both subjects and housewives continuing to carry out their usual tasks. The changes observed seem unlikely to be dilution effects, because there was no change in the serum globulins, cholesterol or triglycerides. Although high doses of beta-blockers can sometimes induce lethargy that reduces ambulation and makes some people supine for long parts of the day, this did *not* happen in the patients studied or they would not have been able to continue with their jobs. They may well have been slowed a little, but they did not complain of tiredness.

H. Keen

Although free fatty acid (FFA) is a major precursor of hepatic triglyceride synthesis, and lowering its blood concentrations might be expected to lower the plasma triglyceride level, there seemed to be absolutely no triglyceride response to the very distinct drop in free fatty acid levels that you demonstrated.

C. W. H. Havard

That is true. There was no change at all in triglyceride levels—which is in accordance with Nilsson's findings (1977), but contrary to Waal-Manning's (1977).

I. H. Mills

In diabetic ketosis, we have shown that continuous naloxone infusion lowers non-esterified fatty acid (NEFA) levels rather dramatically. Since the fall in NEFA and beta-hydroxybutyrate levels do not correlate with the changes in glucose concentration, it may be that endorphins or enkephalins have something to do with control of lipid levels.

D. Leslie

Stubbs *et al.* (1979) found enkephalin analogue had no significant lipolytic activity. When the analogue was infused intravenously, a small degree of lipolysis occurred but this was due to a concomitant rise in growth hormone. No lipolytic activity was demonstrated *in vitro* and, when the analogue was given to hypopituitary patients who did not have a rise in growth hormone, there was no lipolysis.

N. Oakley

Regarding Professor Keen's comment about the disparity between reduced FFA levels and triglyceride levels which remain steady, this may be because the latter is measured in a way that gives no information about triglyceride production or removal rates. There could be quite profound changes in triglyceride turnover without appreciable changes in the circulating level.

Plasma Free Fatty Acids During Squash (Abstract)

M. R. STEPHENS, A. B. DAVIES, R. DOWDLE and A. H. HENDERSON

Department of Cardiology, University Hospital of Wales, Cardiff

With the recent emphasis on "exercise for health", reports of heart attacks during or after recreational exercise have acquired a new importance and, indeed, raise questions of potential personal concern. Although it is difficult to obtain definite data, the acute episode often comes on after rather than during exercise. To investigate the question further, we have conducted some studies on cardiac rhythm during squash playing and have also recorded changes in plasma free fatty acids (FFA) both during and after the game.

Clinical and experimental evidence indicates that high levels of FFA may depress cardiac contraction and cause arrhythmias, probably by increasing the oxygen cost of mechanical work and so inducing or exacerbating any underlying ischaemia. During exercise, increased lipolysis releases FFA and glycerol, the former being used as substrate for muscle work, but rebounding to high levels as soon as work ceases. Little attention has previously been paid to the high levels of FFA during and after a competitive game like squash, or to the possibility that it might contribute to cardiac arrhythmias.

Our observations in fit fasting squash players show that plasma FFA rises slightly during exercise, and that there is an abrupt post-exercise rise to double the pre-exercise levels after 5 min, with an equally rapid fall, followed by a progressive secondary rise in these fasting subjects (Fig. 1). Plasma triglycerides and cholesterol remain normal and glycerol levels follow the predicted changes in lipolytic activity. When the same subjects are exercised to maximum physical capacity on a bicycle ergometer similar changes are seen during exercise, but the post-exercise peak

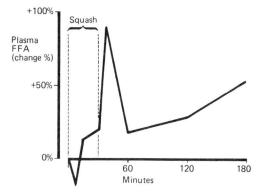

Figure 1. Changes in plasma FFA levels after a game of squash—trained subjects.

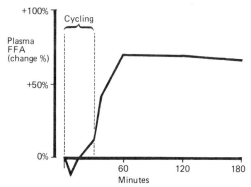

Figure 2. Changes in plasma FFA levels after bicycle ergometry.

is both less pronounced and significantly more prolonged (Fig. 2). This is probably related to the competitive nature of squash and thus to the

The Cardiovascular, Metabolic and Psychological Interface: Royal Society of Medicine International Congress and Symposium Series No. 14, published jointly by Academic Press Inc. (London) Ltd., and the Royal Society of Medicine.

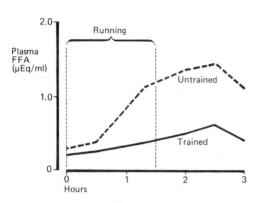

Figure 3. *Changes in plasma FFA levels during running—trained and untrained subjects compared.*

greater activation of the sympathetic system. It is notable that the sinus tachycardia during squash was 200 beats/min compared to 170 during bicycle ergometry.

A post-exercise rise of FFA could therefore contribute to the causation of serious arrhythmias and these can, of course, initiate myocardial infarction. This preliminary study has been carried out on fit volunteers and no arrhythmias were observed. Further studies in unfit subjects may show that FFA can rise to even higher levels (Fig. 3), perhaps even precipitating overt features of ischaemia in subjects with asymptomatic coronary artery disease. It is well known that electrocardiographic evidence of ischaemia and arrhythmias often occur after rather than during exercise testing. There are, of course, many possible explanations for this apparent paradox—of which the post-exercise rise in FFA may be one.

Discussion
M. Carruthers

I do agree with Dr Stephen that more studies are needed of the everyday forms of exercise that people will take up and continue as part of their ways of life. I too am concerned about the exceptionally competitive element in squash. Sometimes there are mishaps because no attention is paid to safety factors by the people taking up this form of sport. Those who are trained and play regularly are not so much at risk but with beginners there is some need to pay attention both to pulse rate and to perceived exertion. People tend to ignore these safety factors when they are caught up in the game.

Secondly, I am interested in what happens after the squash game. Did Dr Stephens' subjects have a shower and if so was it hot or cold? Cold showers can promote noradrenaline release and free fatty acid response, whereas hot showers (if comparable with sauna bathing, which we have studied) can probably produce pulse rates as high as or even higher than those seen to result from adrenaline release during exercise. How did the subjects behave after their game of squash?

M. R. Stephens

They took a warm shower. I cannot explain the profound fall in free fatty acid concentration which suddenly occurs after the early massive rebound, but I agree that the highly competitive nature of this particular game probably has a very important bearing on the physiological changes that are observed.

H. Keen

It might be possible to explain the rise in free fatty acids immediately after exercise on the basis of some observations we made many years ago on oxygen concentration in femoral venous blood immediately after exercise: it rapidly approaches that of arterial blood and we interpreted this as meaning that the muscles through which this blood had flowed were no longer extracting oxygen from it but remained in a state of massive hyperaemia until suddenly washed through by arterial blood. This may also be so of blood loaded with unextracted non-esterified fatty acid, which then gets picked up by the liver or elsewhere.

P. S. Sever

Dr Edelman and I were both struck by your description of the various attributes of squash, which it seems to share with the act of sexual intercourse. Which type of exercise is sexual intercourse, as far as behaviour of the free fatty acids is concerned?

I. H. Mills

The rise in blood pressure during sexual intercourse and orgasm is completely blocked with a beta-blocker. As regards changes in free fatty acid levels, of course the data on people who died in sexual intercourse is not usually published, but quite an appreciable number do die in this way.

P. Bennett

Another important aspect is the taking of drugs by subjects about to engage in strenuous physical exercise, either stimulant drugs by sportsmen or, innocently, by people taking cold cures which contain sympathomimetic agents. I think that this is something which is not sufficiently widely recognized and may contribute to the mortality of sudden physical exercise.

M. Carruthers

In Japan there are more fatalities in away matches than home matches.

G. H. Hall

If as seems likely the free fatty acids are responsible for this, the corollary is that beta-blockers might possibly prevent it. We found that if beta-blockers are taken during extreme exercise the mixed venous blood becomes extremely desaturated—in fact the opposite of what Professor Keen found. There was also a very marked elevation of lactate levels which lasted a long time and made one feel very exhausted.

S. H. Taylor

Dr Stephens, as you were monitoring your squash players by continuous electro-cardiogram, did you see any dysrhythmias and secondly, do you consider that the vagus might well play an important role in the period after exercise?

M. R. Stephens

We did not in fact find any arrhythmias. Obviously, to justify the whole concept that high free fatty acid levels are associated with arrhythmias one would have to find evidence that they occur, but quite clearly one might have to examine as many as 3000 subjects to find just one case, and then this case occurring in this situation would be highly significant. However, it would not be desirable to carry out this sort of observation on people with myocardial ischaemia, and in any case this may not be the right approach, so the concept is certainly not invalidated by our not having come across cases of arrhythmia. We shall continue to watch for them and will also be measuring potassium levels, which we have not done so far.

I. H. Mills

There may be yet another aspect to be considered: that of steroid responses to stress. In an early study the cox of a boat was taken as control but his steroid response to the race turned out to be as great as those of the oarsmen who were doing all the physical work. In other words, there must be in the competitive game a high emotional effect, and I wonder whether this is not playing some part in release of steroids, endorphins and so on.

M. R. Stephens

I quite agree.

Effect of Beta-adrenergic Receptor Blockade on Glucose Homoeostasis in Maturity-onset Diabetes (Abstract)

P. BIGGS

Walsgrave Hospital, Coventry

Beta-adrenergic blocking drugs are now extensively used for the treatment of angina and hypertension. In diabetics, they would be of particular value as it is well known that diabetic patients are prone to cardiovascular diseases. However, their use in diabetics has been less than enthusiastic, mainly because of the fear that they may mask the warning signs of an impending hypoglycaemic attack. This concern may have been exaggerated. Nevertheless, the effect of beta-receptor blocking drugs on carbohydrate metabolism has been difficult to interpret, and the results of studies have been conflicting.

Abramson *et al.* (1966) was the first to report hypoglycaemia in association with the use of beta-blocking drugs. Loubatières *et al.* (1971) demon-

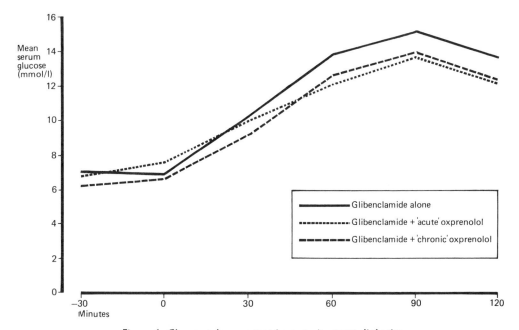

Figure 1. Glucose tolerance test in maturity-onset diabetics.

The Cardiovascular, Metabolic and Psychological Interface: Royal Society of Medicine International Congress and Symposium Series No. 14, published jointly by Academic Press Inc. (London) Ltd., and the Royal Society of Medicine.

strated a fall in blood glucose levels following beta-adrenergic blockade. More recently Newman (1976), and Deacon and Barnett (1976) showed potentiation of insulin-induced hypoglycaemia. On the other hand, Robertson and Porte (1973) showed no effect of beta-blockade on blood glucose.

With respect to insulin, Cerasi *et al.* (1972) showed inhibition of insulin secretion by beta-receptor blockade. Lufkin *et al.* (1971) found that beta-blockade potentiated release of growth hormone (GH), one of the diabetogenic hormones. Thus the combination of increased GH release with inhibition of secretion of insulin may be deleterious to the diabetic, particularly the maturity-onset diabetic with some residual insulin secretion.

To investigate the effect of beta-blockade on glucose homoeostasis in maturity-onset diabetics, we have used two drugs—a non-selective beta-blocker (oxprenolol) and a cardioselective beta-blocker (metoprolol)—on male subjects aged 70 years or less who were well controlled on gliben-clamide, and who were not taking any drugs or

had any diseases likely to affect carbohydrate metabolism.

The patients were admitted to hospital for the study, and their calorie intake was controlled. Each patient was studied by glucose tolerance tests (GTT) and whole-day glucose profiles. The first (control) test was carried out before treatment, the next ("acute") test at the start of beta-blockade, and the final ("chronic") test after 3 weeks' continuous therapy. Blood was taken *via* an indwelling canula for determination of glucose levels by autoanalyser. Five subjects were given oxprenolol (80 mg twice daily) and four meto-prolol (100 mg twice daily) 1 h before GTT or a meal. The findings in five volunteer patients are shown in Figs 1 and 2. Oxprenolol significantly reduced the peak glucose level at 90 min after a 50 g GTT, which occurred after both "acute" ($P < 0.05$) and long-term ($P < 0.1$) therapy. Three weeks' treatment with oxprenolol significantly lowered the blood glucose level in the whole-day profiles measured by area under the curve. Metoprolol had no effect on blood glucose either in the GTT or day profile.

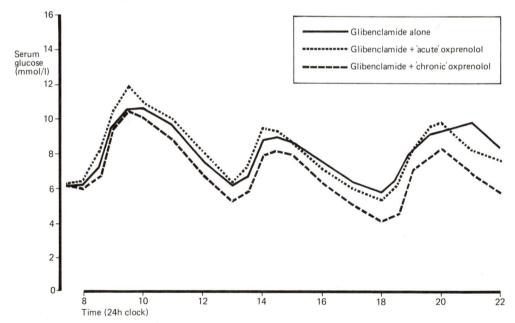

Figure 2. *Mean glucose profile (five volunteers).*

References

Abramson, E. A., Arky, R. A. and Woeber, K. A. (1966). Effects of propranolol on the hormonal and metabolic responses to insulin-induced hypoglycaemia. *Lancet* **2**, 1386.

Cerasi, E., Luft, R. and Efendić, S. (1972). Effect of adrenergic blocking agents on insulin response to glucose infusion in man. *Acta endocrinologica* **69**, 335.

Deacon, S. P. and Barnett, D. (1976). Comparison of atenolol and propranolol during insulin-induced hypoglycaemia. *Brit. med. J.* **2**, 272.

Loubatières, A., Mariani, M. M., Sorel, G. and Savi, L. (1971). The action of β-adrenergic blocking and stimulating agents on insulin secretion. Characterization of the type of β reception. *Diabetologia* **7**, 127.

Lufkin, E. G., Greene, H. L., Meek, J. R. and Herman, R. H. (1971). Adrenergic control of hormone secretion. *Journal of Laboratory & Clinical Medicine* **78**, 820.

Newman, R. J. (1976), Comparison of propranolol, metoprolol, and acebutol on insulin-induced hypoglycaemia. *Brit. med. J.* **2**, 447.

Robertson, R. P. and Porte, D., Jr (1973). Adrenergic modulation of basal insulin secretion in man. *Diabetes* **22**, 1.

Discussion
H. Keen

That is a fascinating and very valuable study. It is interesting to note that so far as the four groups that we challenged with glucose were concerned, the one group which did actually show an improvement in glucose tolerance after oxprenolol was the group taking oral anti-diabetic agents, which makes our findings comparable with yours. There may be some sort of interaction between all anti-diabetic agents and oxprenolol.

Diabetes and Beta-blockade
(Abstract)

P. W. ADAMS

St Mary's Hospital, London

Beta-adrenoceptor blocking agents may impair glucose tolerance and inhibit the rise of glucose and free fatty acid (FFA) following hypoglycaemia or exercise. It has been proposed that the use of cardioselective beta$_1$-blocker agents without membrane-stabilizing and intrinsic sympathomimetric activities should be preferred in diabetic patients as it has been suggested that they might have fewer metabolic side effects.

Purpose of Study

To determine whether the administration of a beta-adrenoceptor blocking agent possessing membrane-stabilizing and intrinsic sympathomimetric activities resulted in adverse effects on carbohydrate and lipid metabolism which would contraindicate its use in diabetics. The effects of oxprenolol have been investigated in two obese subjects and seven untreated diabetics with glucose intolerance ranging in severity from glycosuria to insulin-deficient diabetes.

Methods

The following were measured:
1. diurnal plasma glucose, insulin, FFA, triglyceride (after chylomicron separation) and cholesterol profiles;
2. plasma glucose, insulin, and glucagon responses during a 3 h oral glucose tolerance test (OGTT);
3. plasma glucose and insulin responses following an intravenous bolus injection of 2 μg isoprenaline; and
4. plasma glucose, FFA and glucagon levels during an insulin stress test (IST, 0·15 u/kg).

The patients were then given oxprenolol 80 mg thrice daily for 6 weeks, when the tests were repeated.

Results

The patients' mean weight was not altered significantly between the two tests, apart from one obese patient who lost 4·6 kg. Isoprenaline-stimulated rises in pulse rates were suppressed in six and greatly reduced in three patients, and the insulin responses to isoprenaline abolished in all patients by oxprenolol, indicating adequate beta-blockade.

Fasting plasma glucose levels (FPG) were elevated by oxprenolol in every patient (mean FPG $\pm$ s.e. mean before treatment = 84·8 $\pm$ 6·9 mg/100 ml; during treatment with oxprenolol = 98·4 $\pm$ 11 mg/100 ml: $P < 0.05$), but the fasting insulin levels were unaltered (Fig. 1). The mean diurnal pre-prandial but not the post-prandial plasma glucose levels were also significantly increased during oxprenolol treatment (Fig. 2).

Glucose tolerance test

The mean OGTT glucose levels were significantly elevated during oxprenolol treatment (Fig. 3). This was due to the change in FPG since the assimilation of the oral glucose load was unaltered (incremental glucose area in the diabetics before treatment = 439 $\pm$ 40; with treatment = 504 $\pm$ 27) The mean OGTT insulin levels were slightly

The Cardiovascular, Metabolic and Psychological Interface: Royal Society of Medicine International Congress and Symposium Series No. 14, published jointly by Academic Press Inc. (London) Ltd., and the Royal Society of Medicine.

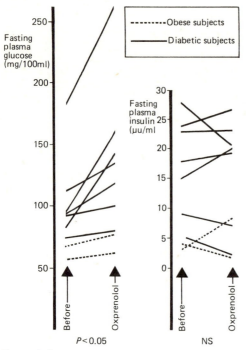

Figure 1. Fasting plasma glucose and insulin levels before and after subjects received oxprenolol.

Insulin stress test

During the IST the fall in plasma glucose was greater (decrement in mg/100 ml before treatment $= -51 \cdot 7 \pm 6 \cdot 7$; and with treatment $= -62 \pm 7 \cdot 1$; $P < 0 \cdot 05$), although the glucose level did not sink so low with oxprenolol (before treatment $= 33 \cdot 9 \pm 5 \cdot 2$ mg/100 ml; and during treatment $= 41 \cdot 6 \pm 5 \cdot 9$ mg/100 ml; $P < 0 \cdot 005$). These effects were related to the prevailing FPG levels since this variable correlated with glucose decrement (before treatment $r = 0 \cdot 591$, NS; during treatment $r = 0 \cdot 954$, $P < 0 \cdot 001$) and the lowest level of plasma glucose (before treatment $r = 0 \cdot 89$, $P < 0 \cdot 01$; during treatment $r = 0 \cdot 964$, $P < 0 \cdot 001$), and there was a strong correlation between the change in FPG and the change in glucose decrement with oxprenolol ($r = 0 \cdot 959$, $P < 0 \cdot 001$). The point at which the latter line of regression intercepted the change in glucose decrement axis (-5 mg/100 ml), and the observation that the fall in plasma glucose expressed as a percentage of FPG was unaltered by oxprenolol (before treatment $= 61\%$ during treatment $= 59\%$), indicate that oxprenolol did not enhance insulin-induced hypoglycaemia.

The glucose recovery following hypoglycaemia (Fig. 5) was not inhibited by oxprenolol (increment before treatment $= 30 \cdot 8 \pm 3 \cdot 1$ mg/100 ml; during treatment $= 32 \cdot 7 \pm 33 \cdot 1$ mg/100 ml). The plasma glucagon levels were unaltered by oxprenolol in both the OGTT and the IST. Oxprenolol reduced the diurnal and IST fasting FFA levels. The changes in fasting FFA and FFA decrement induced by insulin were correlated ($r = 0 \cdot 73$, $P < 0 \cdot 05$) and their relationship suggested that

higher with oxprenolol but the total insulin responses were unaltered (Fig. 4). The corresponding incremental insulin areas in the diabetics were: before treatment $= 369 \cdot 4 \pm 163$; and during treatment $= 393 \cdot 8 \pm 173$. The diurnal insulin responses were also unaltered.

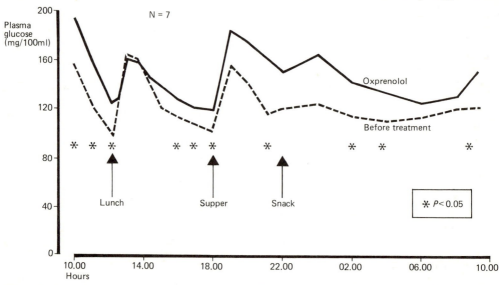

Figure 2. Mean diurnal preprandial but not post-prandial plasma glucose levels were significantly raised by oxprenolol.

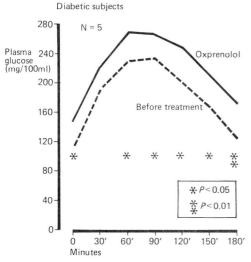

Figure 3. Mean plasma glucose levels during an oral glucose tolerance test were raised during oxprenolol treatment.

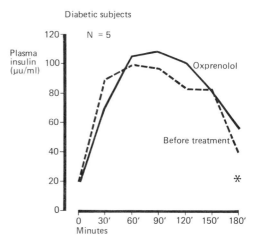

Figure 4. Insulin levels before and during oxprenolol treatment in a glucose tolerance test.

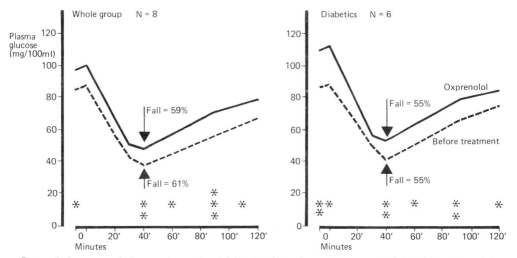

Figure 5. Recovery of plasma glucose level following hypoglycaemia was not inhibited by oxprenolol.

oxprenolol enhanced inhibition of lipolysis by insulin. The FFA recovery following hypoglycaemia was reduced by oxprenolol (FFA increment as a percentage of fasting level before treatment = 82%, during treatment = 51%). The mean diurnal cholesterol levels were unchanged, but the triglyceride levels were significantly elevated in every subject throughout the 24 h by oxprenolol (mean before treatment = $190 \cdot 4 \pm 7 \cdot 8$ mg/100 ml; during treatment = $235 \cdot 7 \pm 3 \cdot 9$ mg/100 ml, $P < 0 \cdot 002$).

Conclusions

The results demonstrate that oxprenolol impairs glucose homoeostasis by elevating the FPG, inhibits basal and stress-induced lipolysis, and elevates triglyceride levels; thus when used in diabetic patients the fasting plasma glucose and triglyceride levels should be closely monitored. The risk of hypoglycaemia with oxprenolol would appear to be minimal.

Discussion
D. Ballantyne

Was the rise in mean triglyceride levels or were there some patients who showed a very mild rise and some who did not show a rise at all, or did they all show a rise?

P. W. Adams

There was a large variation because the patients themselves varied quite widely. One patient, for example, had very marked insulin resistance with enhanced peripheral lipolysis, hyperinsulinaemia and high triglyceride production; such people have high triglyceride levels and this man's showed a marked rise with oxprenolol; others showed less marked rises, but in no case did the level fall.

D. Ballantyne

Did you control the diet during these stages?

P. W. Adams

We attempted outpatient dietary control, to maintain a constant weight. One of the obese patients lost 4·6 kg but there was no change in the mean weight of the patients during the study.

R. J. Jarrett

There is an apparent discrepancy between the results of the last two papers in relation to oxprenolol and diabetics not being treated with oral antidiabetic agents. Dr Biggs stated that all his patients were non-obese, within 120% of standard body weight. Dr Adams mentioned that some of his patients were obese, so obesity is not an explanation of the difference in response between the two groups. This is important because looking at Dr Adams' mean figures the results before oxprenolol would place his patients in the category which is now being defined as impaired glucose tolerance. The mean results with oxprenolol would place them in the category defined as diabetes, so if his results can be extrapolated to the general population, it would make a considerable difference to the numbers of people being diagnosed as diabetic under the new criteria.

P. W. Adams

Yes, it may well do.

H. Keen

I wonder what results would have been obtained if patients had been given placebo tablets for 6 weeks. Do you suppose the fact that you were taking an interest in them and doing something special to them might have altered their behaviour and way of life, and that the changes you saw were attributable to that rather than to the drug?

P. W. Adams

I would have expected their plasma glucose levels to have fallen simply on the basis of an interest being taken in them.

R. W. Elsdon-Dew

In the light of what we have heard, would members of the panel choose a beta-blocker as their choice for the treatment of a diabetic patient with hypertension?

H. Keen

I do use beta-blocking agents to treat hypertesion in diabetics, usually oxprenolol, but increasingly metoprolol, but admittedly more for theoretical than for practical reasons.

C. W. H. Havard

I do not see many diabetics, as this is not my specialty, but I have used metoprolol and have not met any problems with it.

P. Biggs

Neither have I.

P. W. Adams

I also agree. I would use a beta-blocker but, again, would prefer a selective one if only on theoretical grounds.

I. H. Mills

Are there not some data that oxprenolol has some alpha-blocking as well as beta-blocking action?

R. W. Elsdon-Dew

The evidence for that is not very well substantiated and I am not sure that the amount of alpha-blockade which has been described is necessarily relevant to oxprenolol itself.

I. H. Mills

No, but it might be of relevance in patients taking very high doses, as it might affect their response to hypoglycaemia. Such data as there are suggest that both alpha- and beta-adrenergic stimulation are involved in recovery from hypoglycaemia; since people vary in the dose of drug that they require to control their blood pressure, this problem might arise.

R. W. Elsdon-Dew

The amount of alpha-blockade is so small that I do not think it would actually interfere with response to hypoglycaemia.

J. A. Gibson

The last two papers appear to give contradictory results. Could the panel explain this, please?

P. Biggs

I believe my own results are accurate and consistent. I only presented the results in nine subjects, but I have studied a number of others too. I have drawn up over thirty day-profiles and all the subjects show similar effects with oxprenolol. Interestingly we found a marked reduction in insulin secretion but no effect of metoprolol on their glucose levels, which I must admit I find difficult to explain.

In another study, in which we were investigating the effects of D-propranolol, two normal subjects had no insulin secretion whatsoever, as tested during a glucose tolerance test, but their glucose curve remained the same as in the control situation. That again I cannot explain.

I. H. Mills

There was no insulin secretion into the peripheral circulation?

P. Biggs

That is so.

P. W. Adams

Were your subjects studied as in-patients, and did their weight remain constant?

P. Biggs

Yes.

P. W. Adams

Do you think that their diet was better controlled on the ward than it had been when they were outpatients?

P. Biggs

The dietician calculated what their diet, as outpatients, actually was (not necessarily what had been recommended), and from that designed 3 isocaloric meals a day for them which they had for the duration of the study.

P. W. Adams

It is very difficult to ensure that patients' diets are accurately assessed, is it not? We all know the pitfalls of this. So could the difference between your results and ours reflect that your patients, being under controlled conditions for 3 weeks, were subjected to more rigid dietary control than they had been outside? With better diabetic and dietary control, one would expect the fasting plasma glucose level to fall.

P. Biggs

I certainly think the difference may well be due to my subjects having had 2 days' controlled isocaloric diet and the fact that they were in hospital meant that we knew exactly what they were taking at least two days before we studied them.

P. W. Adams

Is 2 days enough? I still think that the critical point may be that your pateints were in hospital, well controlled, while ours were outpatients, although they did not change in weight and so probably did not alter their dietary intake to any significant extent. I tried to explain the elevation of the fasting plasma glucose level by elimination of the peripheral beta effect by oxprenolol, allowing the alpha effect to become predominant in the liver: there is published work to show that this is possible.

I. H. Mills

I think we end up with what is, from the audience's point of view, not a completely satisfactory answer.

P. S. Sever

I am always a little uncertain when I see data presented on small numbers of patients, particularly as shown in the last paper, in which mean values were given on the slides but no error bars nor standard deviations. I would want to know what sort of statistical method was applied to the analysis of those data, because it is very easy to show significant differences using simple Student's t tests but, if the data are not normally distributed, then entirely erroneous conclusions may be arrived at if the appropriate statistical method is not used.

P. W. Adams

Data were logarithmically transformed for analysis; in all instances such transformation led to a parametric distribution appropriate for the statistical method used: that is, the paired Student's t test.

P. Bennett

We have not seen any data on plasma levels of oxprenolol or metoprolol. These can be very variable; oxprenolol, certainly, is a drug which undergoes extensive presystemic elimination and the amount of drug appearing in the systemic circulation depends on how much is removed by the liver. That is what we are concerned about —plasma levels of these drugs.

H. Keen

In our second study, of the response to and recovery from hypoglycaemia, we measured both oxprenolol and metoprolol blood levels but the data have not yet been fully analysed.

C. W. H. Havard

In our study of lipids, we did not measure blood metoprolol levels.

P. Biggs

I did not measure blood levels in my study but one has to be very careful about correlating blood levels with physiological effect.

P. W. Adams

We did not measure the blood levels of oxprenolol, either.

S. H. Taylor

What does the panel consider the clinical pathophysiological significance of their findings to be, particularly as most of our patients with angina and hypertension do not have carbohydrate intolerance?

H. Keen

Without the right sort of study, all one can do is to make what one hopes are reasonably responsible predictions about what might happen. On the basis of our own studies and most of the other studies that I have had access to and read, I would argue that—from the diabetic's point of view, at any rate—there seems to be remarkably little perturbation of metabolism. I am not really impressed by the data on lipid changes which might be supposed to be a risk in terms of long-term development of arterial disease. In the short term, I think there are no very obvious threats to life and health for the diabetic. So far as the non-diabetic is concerned, I am quite convinced that beta-blockers are not diabetogenic agents; that is to say, the minimal effects that they sometimes have on glucose tolerance are very unlikely to add up to anything of clinical significance.

C. W. H. Havard

I really have little to add but if one was giving a hypertensive patient long-term treatment with a beta-blocker, I think it would be wiser to choose one that did not raise cholesterol or triglyceride levels, rather than one that did.

P. W. Adams

Patients could be monitored for major metabolic changes very simply by routine measurement of their fasting plasma glucose and lipid levels, for which no special laboratory facilities are needed. Much experimental work on the effects of beta-blockers on lipolysis has been reported and it has been shown that postprandial hypertriglyceridaemia is accentuated by inhibition of lipoprotein lipase as judged by post-heparin lipolytic activity. I have carried out studies of free-fatty-acid flux in other patients taking oxprenolol and preliminary results indicate inhibition of peripheral lipolysis. This suggests that the rise in serum triglyceride is likely to be due to impaired clearance, supporting the animal work on lipoprotein lipase.

H. Keen

Is there any information yet about the effects of beta-blockade on high-density lipoproteins?

P. W. Adams

I have seen it quoted that beta-blockers do lower high-density lipoprotein levels.

N. Oakley

I would like to return to the apparent discrepancies between Dr Biggs' and Dr Adams' findings. It was gratifying to see that the fasting plasma insulin level was unaltered by beta-blockade: if one follows the concept that Dr Turner in Oxford has been putting forward—that the glucose level achieved in the fasting state is such that the insulin level is appropriate to the maintenance of equilibrium between glucose production and glucose utilization, which is surely characteristic of the patient and his pancreas—then one should indeed find an unchanged insulin level but a slightly different glucose level on beta-blockade. Can I ask Dr Biggs about the effect of beta-blockade on the fasting plasma insulin levels in his study?

P. Biggs

In the results received so far there has been very little difference in fasting insulin levels, certainly no significant difference.

I. H. Mills

Data were presented at the Kinin 1978 conference in Tokyo recently that bradykinin infused into the forearm increases glucose utilization without any changes in insulin levels, and it was postulated that increased blood flow might play a part in this. Does Professor Keen think that beta-blockade can alter glucose levels irrespective of changes in insulin level, which is what we are being asked to believe, by any such phenomenon?

H. Keen

It is fairly apparent from our discussion that there are three areas in which our knowledge is still hazy. First, what is the interaction between the beta-cells of the islets of Langerhans and the liver? We measure insulin levels in the peripheral circulation, and have limited information on possible effects of beta-blockade on uptake or effectiveness of insulin at the liver, or on splanchnic blood flow which may itself influence insulin in the liver: a large part of the effect of insulin on plasma glucose is by way of its effects upon the liver, but we need to know more about this.

The second area is that of the metabolic effects of beta-blockers on peripheral tissue. Asmal and his colleagues in South Africa claim to have demonstrated that when oxprenolol is infused into the brachial artery it has a direct effect on the metabolism of the forearm muscles. They did use fairly large amounts, however, and it may be that this high-dose experiment is not very relevant to what happens during ordinary therapeutic use of the drug.

Finally, there may well be effects in the brain and hypothalamus, especially with regard to some of the fragments of the beta-lipotrophin molecule which exert quite a dramatic influence on peripheral metabolism. A fragment or fragments of that molecule have been shown to influence glucose and insulin metabolism. We have no idea of the possible effect of beta-blockade on that.

B. I. Hoffbrand

If I may return to the effect of beta-blockers on high-density lipoprotein levels: two studies have been reported, both on uncontrolled populations, suggesting that treatment with propranolol may lower high-density lipoprotein levels, but this needs to be investigated under properly controlled conditions.

Then, to come back to the theme of diabetes and beta-blockade, I am sure that many members of the audience feel that there is more to the story than perhaps we have heard from the platform this afternoon. I am particularly sceptical about the relevance of "acute" studies, such as those of Professor Keen, to the problems of long-term treatment with beta-blockade, bearing in mind the differing changes brought about by acute and chronic treatment in other respects, particularly in hypertension. We have a patient with severe hypertension whom we treated with large doses of propranolol and later with diazoxide, which made him diabetic. We therefore treated him with tolbutamide and he then had several acute hypoglycaemic episodes. This is just one case but to us it was clinically a very impressive case indeed and I do feel that there is more to the story.

H. Keen

I am sure there is. As you may know, soon after the introduction of beta-blocking agents, the British Diabetic Association became concerned about the possibility of severe hypoglycaemia occurring in unwarned patients or physicians and ran a fairly comprehensive enquiry through the country, to which there were virtually no positive responses. That is only soft data, I agree, but it must mean that no massive epidemic of hypoglycaemia was occurring. There must be individual variability in response to beta-blockers, as there is to all drugs, but the evidence is that there are no major problems in the use of beta-blockers in diabetic patients.

B. I. Hoffbrand

Certainly our own patient was on particularly large doses of beta-blocker.

I. H. Mills

Perhaps one word of warning ought to be breathed at this point: we do not know much about the part some beta-blockers may play in lowering plasma renin activity. I suspect that there are more aspects of beta-blocking drugs than we are always aware of, and I think that one should not assume from the discussion today that all beta-blockers will be equally safe under all circumstances.

V. B. Whitmarsh

In view of what we have heard, would the panel care to comment upon the recommendation which is usually found in package leaflets for beta-blockers: "diabetic patients on beta-blockade should be treated with caution"?

P. W. Adams

In the light of our finding that oxprenolol raised the fasting plasma glucose in very mild diabetics, care should perhaps be taken in giving these drugs to such patients, but I do think the risks of hypoglycaemia are negligible and have been greatly overstated.

P. Biggs

I agree that diabetics given beta-blockers should be followed up very closely, especially at first, but after perhaps a month or two and if no untoward effects have occurred, then I follow these patients up as I would do any other diabetics.

I. H. Mills

I would agree that one should be very cautious, particularly if it is the first time the patient has been given a beta-blocker, and especially if it is one, the nature of which has not been fully established. If there are no more comments on this aspect, I should like to ask Dr Stephens whether he thinks the rise in fatty acids is really the explanation of the sudden deaths that he mentioned.

M. R. Stephens

This question is crucial, of course. I cannot give the answer but clearly the experimental data are very strong. It is also becoming apparent that the post-exercise phase, when we know that these very massive changes in at least the plasma levels of free fatty acids are occurring, probably is in fact the so-called vulnerable period for ischaemia. Certainly this is an area which needs further study.

D. Ballantyne

The report of the working party of the Royal College of Physicians of London and the British Cardiac Society recommended that after myocardial infarction patients should be encouraged to take up a graded exercise programme but, from what you say, do you think this is a dangerous recommendation?

M. R. Stephens

No, I do not think it is a particularly dangerous recommendation. My own observations here have been confined purely to what I personally consider to be a rather vicious form of exercise, squash, and I think that is extremely different from the sort of exercise that most of us clinicians are going to advise our patients who have just had a coronary to undertake. If one looks purely at the problem of the free fatty acid levels, then clearly the changes that one would expect and the magnitude of change with relatively relaxing exercise is totally different from that seen in squash.

D. Ballantyne

Yes, but on the other hand these patients are presumably at greater risk than the sort of squash-playing subjects whom you are studying.

M. R. Stephens

Yes.

J. P. O'Loughlin

Is the incidence of sudden death during the squash game and shortly afterwards higher than expected? Just as some people may die in their armchair, a certain number might be expected to die during a game of squash, since so many middle-aged people play it, unless of course the game had a positive protective action. Are there any data on an increased incidence and should squash-playing be regarded in the future as a positive risk factor?

M. R. Stephens

I do not have any data on this very important question, but there is no doubt that the metabolic changes that are occurring in very severe exercise like squash are immense nor that many 40-year-old people taking up the game for the first time must have some coronary artery disease.

R. J. Jarrett

All of us in our 40s have some coronary artery disease and I should have thought that the average person with significant coronary artery disease is going to get angina as a warning symptom if the exercise is too much for him, and that the actual risk from what one might call a metabolic death must be very very small indeed. Reverting to the statistics of deaths and coronary artery disease, there have been studies on this in relation to time of day and such occurrences are fairly evenly distributed around the clock, so the actual relationship between sudden deaths and exercise is very small indeed and it would be very hard to prove that squash-playing was a risk factor.

M. R. Stephens

I cannot accept that angina relates particluarly closely to the severity of coronary artery disease or the anatomy; I think it is a highly unreliable phenomenon. I showed just one example of a man of 32 who had a total occlusion of the left coronary artery and played squash for many years—presumably with that—yet had no angina, which illustrates how unreliable this symptom can be in indicating severity of disease.

I. H. Mills

Do members of the panel have any closing remarks they would like to make?

C. W. H. Havard

It would seem to me that most people over the age of 40 are ill-advised to take strenuous exercise. I do not include jogging as a strenuous exercise because I often walk in Regent's Park and overtake many of the joggers I see there!

P. W. Adams

I think that this symposium has shown that we desperately need more studies, larger numbers of patients including diabetics, and perhaps more standardization in our methods of investigation. We should coordinate our attack on the problem.

Personality, Type A Behaviour Pattern and Coronary Heart Disease (Abstract)

RAY H. ROSENMAN

Harold Brunn Institute, San Francisco

The incidence of ischaemic heart disease (IHD) did not begin to be significant until the second decade of the twentieth century, after which rapidly increasing rates of IHD occurred in middle-aged males of the Western world. The "epidemic" accompanied modern civilization, which implied a major causal role of the environment. The background substrate is widely believed to be a habitual excess of saturated fats in the diet and a relatively sedentary life. Individual specificity is ascribed to risk factors, serum cholesterol and HDL levels, magnitude of blood pressure and cigarette smoking being held mainly responsible. Although there is much evidence that each of these contributes to the genesis of coronary atherosclerosis and is a risk factor for emergence of IHD, equally as much evidence has accumulated to show that even when all are fully taken into account, they are simply not sufficient to explain either the twentieth-century epidemic or individual specificity of risk. Indeed, the standard risk factors numerically account for less than half of the incidence of IHD in any given population under prospective study. They also fail to account for major geographic differences in prevalence and incidence of IHD at similar levels of these risk factors. As a number of cogent journal editorials have emphasized recently, the evidence that alteration of these risk factors has reduced the primary or recurring risk of IHD is miniscule compared to the remarkable aura of faith that surrounds concepts of their causal relevance.

Much evidence now strongly indicates that additional factors play a role of great relevance, and that these are associated with the socio-economic and psychosocial stress of modern Western civilization. The victimized subjects usually exhibit certain personality traits and appear to be challenged by the uniquely new twentieth-century stress. There is an interaction of such personality traits with the environment such as to engender the coronary-prone Type A behaviour pattern (TABP).

The concept of causal relevance for IHD of certain personality traits and overt behaviour pattern is not new. It has been emphasized by among others, Osler (1897), the Menningers (1936), Arlow (1945) and Stewart (1950). The TABP person exhibits specific personality traits, with enhanced ambitiousness, aggressiveness and competitiveness that evolves into hostility, and is hard-driving and goal-directed. Such traits do not operate in a vacuum but are "activated" by the twentieth-century challenges. This activation

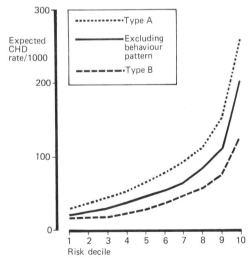

Figure 1. CHD rates/1000 for males aged 39–49 by deciles of estimated risk.

The Cardiovascular, Metabolic and Psychological Interface: Royal Society of Medicine International Congress and Symposium Series No. 14, published jointly by Academic Press Inc. (London) Ltd., and the Royal Society of Medicine.

depends upon the nature of the specific environmental stimuli and challenges that confront the susceptible Type A individual, as well as upon the latter's interpretation of these environmental demands and challenges—hence the response of the coronary-prone Type A person that is characterized by augmented adrenergic discharge. It is from this interaction that the coronary-prone TABP is engendered. Even subjects with lesser Type A personality traits may of necessity often have to comply with the chronic confrontations from which a habitual sense of urgency develops.

The chronic struggle may consist of attempts to do more and more in less and less time, or of repeated conflicts with others. Thus Type As may be preoccupied with deadlines and are usually work-orientated. It should be realized that TABP cannot be equated with stress, stressful situations or distressed symptoms, since it is only the style of response with which Type A individuals confront and try to control their life situations.

TABP is associated with a significantly increased incidence of IHD in our prospective studies, even after full adjustment is made for interactions with other risk factors. The association of TABP with the prevalence and incidence of IHD has now been widely confirmed, with a consistency of findings by many other investigators. Its association with the emergence of a specific disease outcome is well demonstrated, with a biological gradient between the predictor variable and the probability of the emergence of

the disease. A number of relevant mechanisms have been shown to mediate between the predictor variable and the disease, and there is confirmation from experimental animal studies.

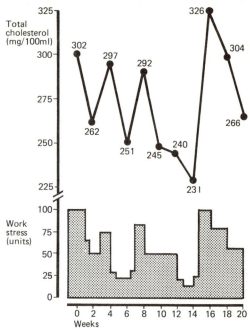

Figure 2. Serum cholesterol levels related to work stress as estimated by an accountant.

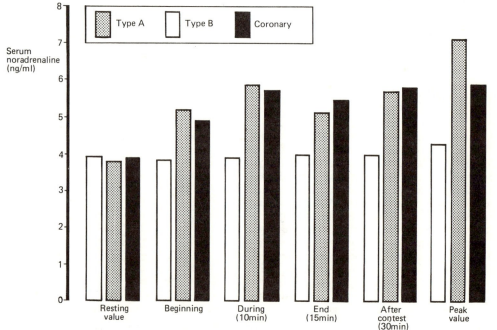

Figure 3. Serum noradrenaline responses to challenge in Types A and B and in coronary patients.

References and Bibliography

Arlow, J. A. (1945). Identification mechanisms in coronary occlusion. *Psychosom. Med.* **7**, 195.

Jenkins, C. D. (1978). Behavioral risk factors in coronary artery disease. *Ann. Rev. Med.* **291**, 543–562.

Menninger, K. A. and Menninger, W. C. (1936). Psychoanalytic observations in cardiac disorders. *Amer. Heart J.* **11**, 10.

National Heart, Lung and Blood Institute (1977). Proceedings of the Forum on Coronary-Prone Behavior, June 1977. DHEW Publication No. (NIH) 78-1451, National Institutes of Health, Bethesda, MD.

Osler, W. (1897). *Lectures on angina pectoris and allied states.* New York, Edinburgh and London.

Rosenman, R. H. and Friedman, M. (1974). Neurogenic factors in the pathogenesis of coronary heart disease. *Med. Clin. N. Amer.* **58**, 269–279.

Stewart, I. McD. G. (1950). Coronary disease and modern stress. *Lancet* **2**, 867.

Discussion
G. S. MacGregor

Doctors, when confronted by disease they do not understand such as scurvy, tuberculosis and general paralysis of the insane, have often blamed stress or arousal. In W. J. Mickle's book "General Paralysis of the Insane" (Mickle, 1880), there is a perfect description of a Type A businessman in a "tranquil" nineteenth-century setting: "the life-long struggles, chagrins and heart burnings, accompanying the modern conflict for existence, for place, power and prestige . . . all conduce to general paralysis". Whilst control of arousal may have been an appropriate if unrealized primary preventive measure in general paralysis of the insane, I wonder how important control of stress and arousal, or modification of Type A personality will be in preventing premature vascular disease, as judged by many previous historical examples?

R. H. Rosenman

We do know most of the factors involved in the pathogenesis of coronary atherosclerosis, even if we cannot yet fit the jigsaw puzzle together perfectly. The roles of dietary and serum lipids, blood pressure, cigarette smoking and Type A behaviour (probably operating through the adrenergic nervous system) are all known, and it is difficult to believe that many important additional new factors will be found. However, since atherogenesis is accelerated by any factor that either damages the coronary arterial intima or accelerates the deposition of lipid into the damaged intima, so additional factors might be found that influence either of these two mechanisms.

G. S. MacGregor

Fifty years ago many doctors emphasized the role of emotion and stress in predisposing towards tuberculosis. However, this is no longer of therapeutic importance because there are now specific drugs for tuberculosis. Therapeutic efforts to modify stress and personality were not very successful in treating tuberculosis; I wonder how successful they will be in treating and preventing premature vascular disease?

R. H. Rosenman

I believe that the incidence of tuberculosis began to decline before any antituberculosis drugs became available. I cannot speak about the role of stress in tuberculosis but it has been convincingly shown that certain aspects of twentieth-century modern stress play a role in the causation of coronary atherosclerosis and, accordingly, in contributing significantly to the incidence of ischaemic heart disease. Such factors interact with other causal agents, including serum cholesterol and blood-pressure level. It is now established that the central nervous system plays a role in atherogenesis: we should try to find out precisely what this mechanism is, so that we can prevent damage to the coronary arteries.

I. H. Mills

Many of the points that have been made have a relationship to known factors in renal physiology. I am quite convinced that the increased adrenergic drive and release of noradrenaline are important. In a paper we will be presenting to the Physiological Society next week we shall make the point that, at any level of the renin-angiotensin system, increased noradrenaline secretion decreases kallikrein release and sodium excretion. There is increasing evidence that in essential hypertension the low kallikrein is of importance. The techniques which increase kallikrein released by the kidney, some of which goes into the urine and some into the circulation, do tend to lower blood pressure.

As regards the point you made about potassium, some years ago we demonstrated that there are a number of conditions in man in which potassium has a very good natriuric action. It decreases sodium re-absorption in the proximal tubule and this delivers a greater sodium and chloride load at the macula densa which is known to change renin output, so that potassium can be shown to have a direct hormonal effect in that respect.

It is also interesting that in patients whom we have treated with tricyclic antidepressants we have sometimes seen quite striking falls in blood pressure, sufficient in some cases to cause them to collapse through postural hypotension. I believe that some of the central factors affecting blood pressure can sometimes be influenced by the drugs we use.

Lastly, on the question of potassium and diuretics, the fashion today is for additional potassium to be prescribed for patients being given potassium-losing diuretics, but this is not a very effective way of maintaining serum potassium and total body potassium. The potassium-sparing diuretics such as triamterine, which is not a very powerful diuretic, maintain body potassium much more effectively.

R. H. Rosenman

I certainly agree with your comments about potassium. This is one of the several reasons why I prefer to treat sustained hypertension with the smallest amount of diuretic agent that is effective and, almost invariably, avoid a larger dosage of diuretic by adding an adrenergic blocker. I believe it is very important to add an adrenergic blocker to the therapeutic regimen given to almost every patient who is being treated for hypertension. If the blood pressure does not respond to the combination of a modest dosage of diuretic and a modest dosage of adrenergic blocker, then I prefer to add a vasodilator. The choice of vasodilator depends upon whether one seeks arteriolar vasodilatation or whether one seeks to reduce after-load, in which event prazosin would be preferable because it also induces venous dilation.

J. B. Edelman

Until recently, most of us had assumed blood pressure was higher in the evening than in the morning, but recently we have been subjected to a battery of 24-h bloodpressure studies and, surprisingly, some of these have shown that the blood pressure is lower at 5.00 p.m. than it is at 9.00 a.m. Would you like to comment on that?

R. H. Rosenman

To learn about any individual's blood pressure, repeated measurements should be taken and considered in relation to both antecedent and concurrent life situations, as well as the individual's responses to these situations. As emphasized by Professor Mill's paper, we do have cognitive and other coping responses to life situations which are concurrent with environmental challenges and which therefore have considerable relevance to the level of the blood pressure at any given moment. In a recent editorial, Dr Pickering pointed out that high and low levels of blood pressure differ by as much as 100% in most persons during the course of the day.

P. J. Bourdillon

The original Framingham survey predicted less than half the mortality of coronary artery disease. When the Type A figures are included, how much of the mortality is explained?

R. H. Rosenman

Epidemiological studies have uncovered relationships between the incidence of ischaemic heart disease and a variety of prospective risk factors. However, because of associations amongst such factors, it appears essential to analyse them in an adequate multivariate context. Multivariate risk analysis is motivated by the need for methods that assess the direct predictive strength associated with each member of a cluster of inter-related risk factors. For example, one important cluster in prediction of ischaemic disease consists of systolic and diastolic blood pressures. With univariate analysis, each measure is examined separately for relation to incidence of ischaemic disease and both show significant predictability. However, only multivariate risk analysis provides a method for determining whether both measures have direct predictability for disease, or whether one appears as a predictor in the univariate sense, wholly or in part, because of its association with the other.

The most widely used model for multivariate analysis has been the multiple logistic risk model. The essence of the multiple risk analysis is to examine changes of risk with varying levels of one factor at various fixed levels of the remaining factors. When many factors are being considered, a traditional method for multiple risk analysis based on cross-tabulation is not feasible. Erratic results occur because too few cases of ischaemic disease must be distributed over too many risk subgroups. Instead, multiple risk analysis can be approached with use of risk models that are being used with increasing frequency in research studies, most notably with the multiple logistic risk model.

The results of such statistical analyses in the Western Collaborative Group Study have been published (Brand *et al.*, 1976; Rosenman *et al.*, 1976). These articles discuss the use of multivariate analysis by this technique and show that the multiple logistic risk model imposes definite constraints on the risk patterns that can emerge from data analysis. The results of the analysis indicated that substantial risk for ischaemic disease was directly associated with the Type A behaviour pattern and that Type A behaviour does not diminish as a risk factor in older compared to younger men. Despite its prevalence and apparent pathogenic force, the addition of the behaviour pattern to the logistic risk equation adds little improvement to effectiveness and efficiency of selection of ischaemic heart disease cases, but it appears that similar results can be expected for any of the traditional risk factors when assessed as a last addition to a list of other relevant risk factors. However, Type A behaviour has been reported to have an additional indirect risk component that operates through elevation of traditional risk factors but, alone, to account for approximately one third of the numerical incidence of ischaemic heart disease in the Western Collaborative Group Study.

P. J. Bourdillon

I gather these techinques are intended to reduce the residual variance of predictors in assessing final outcome. Every variable that is of use when considered independently of the others should reduce residual variance. If Type A behaviour is taken into account as an additional factor in considering the data from the original Framingham study, to what exent does it reduce that variance?

R. H. Rosenman

About one-third of the incidence of ischaemic heart disease is accounted for by the Type A behaviour pattern, in both younger and older middle-aged males.

G. Sartory

Can all behaviour be classified as Type A or Type B or are these patterns the extremes between which there is a whole range of intermediate behaviour?

R. H. Rosenman

We prefer to assess the behaviour pattern by the structured interview (Rosenman *et al.*, 1964). It is most useful to assess most individuals as exhibiting either Type A or Type B behaviour patterns, but a few cannot be grouped in this way and to these we assign a special designation—Type X. I am not at all certain that this represents a true continuum, although our own survey does provide a continuum of scores both for the global behaviour pattern as well as for several facets of behaviour that can be found within the global pattern. The Type A and Type B designations do not refer to extreme groups of the population but are applicable to any population that can be found anywhere.

B. I. Hoffbrand

I was not quite clear whether the relationships which have been shown between personality and coronary artery disease on the one hand, and blood cholesterol and coronary artery disease on the other, were in fact independent relationships. In other words, was the analysis univariate?

R. H. Rosenman

The published studies which investigated the relationships between Type A behaviour and the angiographic degree of basic coronary atherosclerosis also included studies of all of the standard risk factors. The data were analysed in each instance by multivariate analysis and accordingly showed a very significant relationship between Type A behaviour and the basic degree of coronary atherosclerosis, after adjustments were made fully for interaction with all other risk factors.

B. I. Hoffbrand

As regards systolic blood pressure, although the relationships you have mentioned are very well recognized and accepted, no one to my mind has yet shown that reduction of systolic blood pressure alone in fact preserves life or prevents strokes and coronaries: a cause-and-effect relationship has not yet been demonstrated. In fact, when we treat diastolic blood pressure, we are treating systolic blood pressure as well, as the two are very closely correlated, but the evidence is not at all persuasive that isolated systolic hypertension is causally related. It probably reflects established arterial disease, and this perhaps also relates to the cold pressor test. There, although the central nevous system is clearly involved, what one is measuring is an expression of the cardiovascular events, the cardiac output and the state of the elastic blood vessels, the great arteries. What do we know about the systolic blood pressure rise in relation to personality? How is it produced? Is it due to increased cardiac output and is this neurologically determined, or is it due to having rather more rigid aortas?

Lastly, I think it is fallacious to argue that the stress of life is an aetiological agent peculiar to our own times: I am sure that there was plenty of stress in former times too.

R. H. Rosenman

There is substantial evidence that systolic blood pressure is not only associated with coronary atherosclerogenesis but is also a risk factor for ischaemic heart disease. In recent years an increasing number of workers have confirmed the strength of this association and raised the question whether the systolic blood pressure is of greater pathogenicity than the diastolic blood pressure.

The relationships of systolic blood pressure to central nervous system activity have been well studied only recently, and increasing attention is being paid to the differences between blood pressure measurements made in the resting state and those made under everyday living conditions, some of which can be mimicked by determining the blood pressure during interviews, cold pressor tests, cognitive tasks and so forth. In every instance in which this relationship has been studied, it was found that Type A and Type B subjects exhibit no differences in mean blood pressure levels or in the prevalence of hypertension but that Type A subjects do show greater rises of systolic blood pressure in response to cold pressor tests, cognitive challenge tasks and even during the structured interview used to assess Type A behaviour pattern.

As regards the question of stress in other ages and in other cultures, I am sure that various stresses also prevailed during the time of Shakespeare, but were quite different from the uniquely new stress which we encounter in twentieth-century urban living—for example, the stress imposed by driving on freeways; physicians having to visit their offices and several hospitals in the course of each day, and, in general, the stress imposed by the pace and other aspects of our twentieth-century environment.

S. H. Taylor

There seems to be some confusion over the haemodynamic origins of the arterial pressure. The *mean* arterial pressure is the ultimate reflection of the volume of blood in the arterial system in relation to its capacity. The *diastolic* pressure is a reflection of the overall systemic vascular resistance. The *systolic* pressure is, in ascending order of importance, a reflection of the elasticity of the aorta and large arteries, the stroke volume and the speed of the left ventricular contraction. The latter is medicated through the inotropic beta-adrenoceptors in the left ventricle. Thus, during sympathetic stimulation such as exercise, the increase in systolic pressure closely follows the increase in heart rate, and both are equally attenuated by beta-blocking drugs.

I. H. Mills

On the last point, it is commonly believed that girls with anorexia nervosa are under a considerable amount of stress, and the patients themselves think so too. Many of them have blood pressures of 90/50 mmHg, even those who never vomit. When they are fed, it is striking that their pulse rate goes up to about 110–120 beats/min but their blood pressure stays at 90/50 mmHg. From the point of view of stress, it may be the patients who are *not* showing the effects of stress who are suffering most.

Dr Jim Henry's work on producing hypertension in mice has been mentioned; he was one of the United States Air Force team who trained the chimpanzees studied during flight in space capsules. The animals were trained to be highly predictable in pressing the right knob or lever at the right time and Henry showed that all the chimpanzees that were successfully trained became markedly hypertensive. I think it is also true of humans: the individuals who can concentrate and get on with the job effectively, without outwardly showing the effects of stress, in fact are the ones who are suffering most. I am not quite sure yet whether any other factor than Type A behaviour can be used to assess that kind of response.

R. H. Rosenman

Air traffic controllers have been shown to develop over the years a prevalence of hypertension which is substantially greater than that found in other subjects who served as controls. The greatest health change occurred in those who initially conformed more closely to Type A and who were in the best physical and emotional health at the outset of their work. Perhaps the explanation is that Type A individuals, who really enjoy their work and derive much satisfaction and pleasure from it, may occasionally "dive" into their work at such an enhanced pace that it engenders too much adrenergic output too much of the time, with the result that changes in their health are more marked.

W. H. Newnham

If I may revert to the concept of scurvy as a stress disorder, as Dr MacGregor suggested: in fact the condition was believed to be due to the miasma or bad atmosphere in the old ships. Dr MacGregor also mentioned tuberculosis in this context and this fits in very well with what Dr Rosenman has been saying. In Leicester, where I work, we have a very high immigrant population of Asians from Kenya and Uganda who were screened on their arrival in this country a few years ago but now, after 4 to 7 years in Leicester, have an appallingly high incidence of tuberculosis. This increased incidence of tuberculosis could be compared with the increased incidence of coronary heart disease which occurs where there are increased population pressures.

Finally, I agree with Professor Mills about the benefits of antidepressants: over the last 13 years I have seen many patients with depression who on admission were taking antihypertensive drugs; after electroplexy to cure their depression not one has needed antihypertensive drugs on discharge from hospital.

References

Brand, R. J., Rosenman, R. H., Sholtz, R. I. and Friedman, M. (1976). *Circulation* **53,** 348.

Mickle, W. J. *General Paralysis of the Insane.* London: H. K. Lewis (1880) pp. 88 and 108.

Rosenman, R. H., Friedman, M., Strauss, R. *et al.* (1964) *Journal of the American Medical Association,* **189,** 15.

Rosenman, R. H., Brand, R. J., Sholtz, R. I. and Friedman, M. (1976). *American Journal of Cardiology* **37,** 903.

Beta-blockers in the Treatment of Anxiety: Further Clinical Experience (Abstract)

J. R. HAWKINGS

North Tees General Hospital,
Stockton-on-Tees

This paper describes the continuation of a clinical study of beta-adrenergic blockade in the treatment of morbid anxiety, the early results of which have already been reported (Hawkings, 1978). The cases studied comprise all the patients under my care in whom treatment by beta-blockade was started for this purpose between Janaury 1st 1971 and July 30th 1978. During this period beta-blockers were prescribed in 510 cases, oxprenolol being used in about three-quarters and pro-pranolol, with one or two exceptions, in the remainder. This report therefore concerns an additional 142 patients seen meanwhile, most of whom received oxprenolol.

The procedure followed was exactly as described earlier, patients being classified by clinical diagnosis into 4 subgroups ("mental anxiety", "phobic anxiety", "anxiety with depression" and "physical anxiety"), as well as being rated on the Hamilton 14-point Anxiety Scale when entering the study and then, at the end of 3 months or when beta-blockade was discontinued, whichever was the earlier, re-assessed as clinically improved or not clinically

Table 1
Outcome of beta-blocker therapy by clinical diagnosis

	Mental anxiety	Phobic anxiety	Anxiety with depression	Physical anxiety	Total
Total	139	123	95	153	510
Treatment abandoned (not tolerated)	15	11	7	15	48
Treatment continued	124	112	88	138	462
Condition improved	78	63	50	118	309
Condition not improved	46	49	38	20	153

Table 2
Response to beta-blocker therapy at 3 months

Improved	309	117 Treatment completed
		192 Treatment continuing
Not improved	153	52 Treatment interrupted
		101 Treatment discontinued

improved, and simultaneously re-rated on the Hamilton Anxiety Scale.

The incidences of intolerance, clinical diagnostic distribution and overall Hamilton Scale Scores are broadly similar to those for the patients already reported upon. The strategy adopted earlier of supplementing pre-existing medication with beta-blockers before withdrawing it, rather than substituting beta-blockers directly, had been

The Cardiovascular, Metabolic and Psychological Interface: Royal Society of Medicine International Congress and Symposium Series No. 14, published jointly by Academic Press Inc. (London) Ltd., and the Royal Society of Medicine.

Table 3
Response in 462 patients completing treatment

Hamilton anxiety scale factors	Before treatment Total scores per factor	% of maximum score possible	Rank	After treatment Total scores per factor	% of maximum score possible	Rank
Maximum score possible per factor	1,848	100		1,848	100	
1. Anxiety	1,262	68·29	4	445	24·08	10
2. Tension	1,585	85·76	2	340	18·39	13
3. Fears	878	47·51	10	575	31·11	4
4. Insomnia	597	32·30	13	510	27·59	6
5. Concentration	634	34·30	12	466	25·22	9
6. Depression	455	24·62	14	336	18·18	14
7. Somatic muscular	1,222	66·12	3	344	18·61	11
8. Somatic sensory	918	49·67	8	578	31·27	3
9. Cardiovascular	1,648	89·17	1	344	18·61	11
10. Respiratory	1,103	59·68	5	505	27·32	7
11. Gastrointestinal	809	43·77	11	468	25·32	8
12. Genitourinary	885	47·88	9	748	40·47	2
13. Autonomic	920	49·78	7	939	50·81	1
14. Interview	937	50·70	6	525	28·40	5
Sum of scores	13,853			7,123		
Average score per patient	29·98	53·54		15·42	27·53	

Table 4
Hamilton anxiety scale scores for individual factors in clinically improved and clinically not improved patients treated by beta-blockade

Hamilton anxiety scale factors	Patients clinically improved Before treatment Score	%	After treatment Score	%	Patients not clinically improved Before treatment Score	%	After treatment Score	%
Maximum possible score per factor	1236	100	1236	100	612	100	612	100
1. Anxiety	793	64·16	99	8·01	469	76·63	346	56·64
2. Tension	1184	95·79	75	6·07	401	65·52	265	43·30
3. Fears	556	44·98	255	20·63	322	52·61	320	52·29
4. Insomnia	346	27·99	263	21·28	251	41·01	247	40·36
5. Concentration	353	28·56	211	17·07	281	45·92	255	41·66
6. Depression	246	19·90	125	10·11	209	34·15	211	34·48
7. Somatic muscular	893	72·25	74	5·99	329	53·76	270	44·12
8. Somatic sensory	576	46·60	230	18·61	342	55·88	348	56·86
9. Cardiovascular	1189	96·20	96	7·77	459	75·00	248	40·52
10. Respiratory	660	53·40	101	8·17	443	72·39	404	66·01
11. Gastrointestinal	581	47·01	230	18·61	228	37·25	238	38·89
12. Genitourinary	553	44·74	427	34·55	332	54·25	321	52·45
13. Autonomic	560	45·31	564	45·63	360	58·82	375	61·27
14. Interview	607	49·11	152	12·30	330	53·92	373	60·95
Total	9097		2902		4756		4221	
Average	29·44	52·57	9·39	16·77	31·08	55·51	27·59	49·27

Table 5
Magnitude of change of Hamilton anxiety scale
factors during treatment with a beta-blocker

Anxiety scale factor (in order of reduced prevalence)	Percentage reduction
Cardiovascular	70·56
Tension	67·37
Somatic muscular	47·51
Anxiety	44·21
Respiratory	32·36
Interview	22·30
Gastrointestinal	18·45
Somatic sensory	18·40
Fears	16·40
Concentration	9·08
Depression	6·44
Genitourinary	7·41
Insomnia	4·71
Autonomic	−1·03
Average	26·01

Table 7
Differences between the pre-treatment scores
(expressed as percentages) in "improved" and
"unimproved" patients

Anxiety scale factor in diminishing order of prevalence	Difference (%)
Tension	+30·27
Cardiovascular	+21·20
Somatic muscular	+18·49
Gastrointestinal	+9·76
Fears	−1·63
Interview	−4·81
Somatic sensory	−9·28
Genitourinary	−9·51
Anxiety	−12·47
Insomnia	−13·02
Autonomic	−13·51
Depression	−14·25
Concentration	−17·36
Respiratory	−18·99

justified by results and was therefore continued in this part of the trial. Similarly, the previous retrospective comparative analysis of results with those in a group of matched patients treated with benzodiazepines, both as regards general efficacy and more particularly drug dependence, had so convincingly favoured treatment with beta-blockers that further comparison of these responses was thought unnecessary.

However, the greater number of patients

Table 6
Magnitude of change in Hamilton anxiety scale factors during treatment by beta-blockade in patients
judged "improved" and "not improved"

"Improved"		"Not improved"	
Anxiety scale factor in order of reduced prevalence	Reduction %	Anxiety scale factor in order of reduced prevalence	Reduction %
Tension	89·72	Cardiovascular	34·48
Cardiovascular	88·43	Tension	22·22
Somatic muscular	66·26	Anxiety	20·09
Anxiety	56·15	Somatic muscular	9·64
Respiratory	45·23	Respiratory	6·38
Interview	36·81	Concentration	4·26
Gastrointestinal	28·40	Genitourinary	1·80
Somatic sensory	27·99	Insomnia	0·65
Fears	24·35	Fears	0·32
Concentration	11·42	Depression	0·33
Genitourinary	10·19	Somatic sensory	0·98
Depression	9·79	Gastrointestinal	−1·64
Insomnia	6·71	Autonomic	−2·45
Autonomic	−0·32	Interview	−7·03
Average	35·80	Average	6·24

studied has now made possible a more detailed analysis of the relevance of the various factors rated on the Hamilton Scale which had earlier simply been used to divide the case material into a "psychic" and a "somatic" group. Tables 1–7 show the total scores and percentages for each factor at the beginning and conclusion of treatment. These indicate the overall profile of the case population under study, the change in that profile brought about by treatment and the magnitude of that change both generally and in respect of each factor. The material is reanalysed after division into the "clinically improved" and "unimproved" groups and these two subpopulations are compared, both with regard to the nature, direction and magnitude of change effected by treatment, and also with regard to the prevalence of each factor in the two subpopulations at the outset of the treatment as potential predictors of a favourable or unfavourable response. These data indicate the importance of cardiovascular tension and somatic muscular tension both as predictors of a favourable response and as contributors to that response.

Reference

Hawkings, J. (1978). Clinical experience with beta-adrenergic blockade in psychiatric practice. *In* "A Therapeutic Approach to the Psyche via the Beta-adrenergic System": Proceedings of a Symposium held during the VIth World Congress of Psychiatry, Hawaii, August 1977. (P. Kielholz, Ed.) pp 53–59. Bern: Huber.

Discussion
P. G. F. Nixon

In about 90% of cardiovascular patients who present with arrhythmias, hypertension or coronary syndromes, the disorder is brought about by the hyperarousal and exhaustion which results from their being compelled to deal with too much information, particularly novel or complex information, and without the benefit of habituation produced by previous experience. Now, I am most reluctant to give these people drugs which might reduce their coping ability. I am most reluctant to use any drug not cleared for high performance duties by the RAF, and the Institute of Aviation has not cleared beta-blockers for use in pilots, who require unimpaired cortical performance. Has Dr Hawkings tested his beta-blockers for their effects on performance in, say, car-drivers, and in his patients whose livelihood depends upon information handling?

J. R. Hawkings

No, and neither has anyone else, as far as I know. Of course in the kind of context in which this study was carried out it would have been quite impossible to do that.

P. G. F. Nixon

So you may be creating a public danger?

J. R. Hawkings

My excuse would be that I am protecting these patients from benzodiazapines, which I think are much more of a public danger; indeed one could say that the main success of the trial is that patients have been protected from being on benzodiazapine drugs long enough for them to get better.

P. G. F. Nixon

I am not here to defend the benzodiazepines.

M. Lader

In fact work has been done on the effect on performance of beta-blockers, both in normal subjects and in patients, using a wide variety of laboratory tests, though admittedly not under real-life conditions. These tests show that benzodiazepines—say, diazepam 2 mg—do affect performance, whereas the beta-blockers are devoid of activity in these tests.

P. G. F. Nixon

Would these results convince the Royal Air Force of the safety of using these drugs?

M. Lader

The Air Force may be very cautious in their recommendations here.

P. G. F. Nixon

So am I.

I. H. Mills

I would like to reiterate the views that Dr Hawkings has expressed about the benzo-diazepines. As I remarked yesterday, the striking thing in my experience is that people who have neuro-endocrine disturbances never seem to have them put right by benzodiazepines, whereas very frequently quite gross disturbances are corrected by tricyclic antidepressants. I am encouraged now to think that perhaps we ought to test the effect of beta-blockers to find out whether they too are helpful here. Incidentally, with regard to the point made by Dr Nixon, the less sedative tricyclic anti-depressants such as nortriptyline have been shown in a number of my patients to cure their anxiety state and make them more efficient at controlling high-speed apparatus at their work, whereas it is well established, of course, that benzodiazepines reduce efficiency.

J. R. Hawkings

I would totally agree with that.

The Effects of Oxprenolol on Pistol Shooting Under Stress (Abstract)

L. C. ANTAL and **C. S. GOOD**

Cressington Park, Liverpool

In stressful situations excessive sympathetic drive may cause anxiety and impair performance (James *et al.*, 1977). Pistol shooting gives an objective measurement of performance under reproducible conditions. Accuracy tends to fall during the stress of competition shooting compared to that in training.

To determine if a skilled task performed under stress could be improved by oxprenolol and to monitor subjective, cardiovascular and metabolic changes, volunteers from the British National Pistol-shooting Squad were studied whilst competing for entry to the British team. The design was a double-blind, within-subject comparison of single oral doses of oxprenolol and placebo. Each weekend of the trial oxprenolol was given on one

Table 1
Comparison of mean standing blood pressure and heart rate before shooting

	Systolic blood pressure (mmHg)		Diastolic blood pressure (mmHg)		Heart rate (beats/min)	
	Oxprenolol	Placebo	Oxprenolol	Placebo	Oxprenolol	Placebo
Slow fire (Oxprenolol 40 mg or placebo)	125	130	82	84	72	84
P	0·028		0·304		<0·001	
Slow fire (Oxprenolol 80 mg or placebo)	118	122	80	82	75	84
P	0·007		0·271		<0·001	
Rapid fire (Oxprenolol 40 mg or placebo)	119	129	82	83	71	81
P	0·001		0·273		<0·001	

The Cardiovascular, Metabolic and Psychological Interface: Royal Society of Medicine International Congress and Symposium Series No. 14, published jointly by Academic Press Inc. (London) Ltd., and the Royal Society of Medicine.

day and placebo on the other in random order, the order being reversed the following weekend. Subjects were not allowed any other drugs, or alcohol, tobacco or caffeine preparation except tea from midnight until the day's study was complete. Immediately before and after shooting, subjects rated their nervousness, concentration and well-being. Their blood pressure and heart rate were measured after standing at ease for 2 min. (Table 1). The heart rate was taken after the blood pressure to avoid possible bias in reading the blood pressure. Side effects were recorded. Venous blood was withdrawn for lipid and catecholamine assay. Urine samples were collected for estimation of catecholamines.

In the first part of the trial the effects of a single oral dose given before a slow-fire match with air pistols was studied. Oxprenolol 40 mg was compared to placebo at the first 2 weekends and oxprenolol 80 mg was compared to placebo at the second 2 weekends. Each subject had to fire 10 sighting and 40 competition shots, giving a maximum score of 400.

In the second part the effect of 40 mg oxprenolol was compared with that of placebo in a rapid-fire match using 0·22 pistols. Each subject shot 30 rounds with timed target exposures, giving a maximum score of 300.

Ten subjects shot in both the slow- and rapid-fire studies. The heart rate was continuously monitored during shooting. Investigators were

the same for each part of the trial. Analysis of variance was used to determine effects due to treatment, day, weekend and volunteer.

During slow fire the mean target score of subjects taking oxprenolol 40 mg was 2·9 points above the mean of those taking placebo; this was statistically significant (Table 2). Thirteen subjects shot better when taking oxprenolol 40 mg, 7 improving their scores by more than 5 points. Five shot worse when taking oxprenolol 40 mg, but in only one case did the score deteriorate by more than 5 points.

When oxprenolol 80 mg was taken, the mean score was 3·4 points above the mean for placebo-takers. Sixteen subjects shot better when taking oxprenolol 80 mg; of these 2 showed a massive improvement. Four subjects scored better when taking placebo, though only one did so by more than 5 points.

Further analysis of the scores showed that the number of "wild" shots (i.e. shots outside the "9" ring) significantly decreased with oxprenolol 40 mg and 80 mg compared to placebo.

During rapid-fire shooting there was no evidence of a statistically significant drug effect on target score although the mean score for oxprenolol-takers was marginally better than the mean for placebo-takers.

With 80 mg oxprenolol nervousness before slow fire was significantly reduced. During slow fire, concentration and well-being were rated as

Table 2
Comparison of mean target scores during pistol shooting

	No. of subjects	Drug effect		Day effect		Weekend	
		Oxprenolol	Placebo	Saturday	Sunday	1	2
Slow fire (Oxprenolol 40 mg or placebo)	18	367·9	365·0	366·0	366·9	365·4	367·5
P		0·041		0·523		0·126	
Slow fire (Oxprenolol 80 mg or placebo)	20	368·7	365·3	365·5	368·5	367·9	366·1
P		0·008		0·018		0·138	
Rapid fire (Oxprenolol 40 mg or placebo)	22	283·4	282·9	282·4	283·8	282·5	283·7
P		0·794		0·444		0·452	

Maximum scores: slow fire, 400; rapid fire, 300.

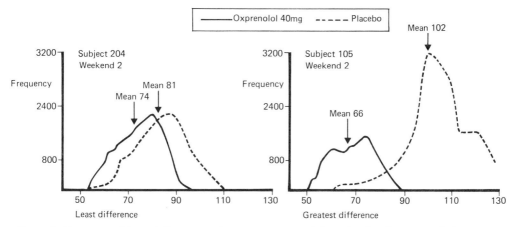

Figure 1. *Greatest and least differences in heart rate, oxprenolol vs placebo, during pistol-shooting— slow fire.*

significantly better with oxprenolol 80 mg and there was a trend in favour of oxprenolol.

During rapid fire, concentration and well-being were rated slightly better with placebo.

Heart rate and systolic pressure were significantly reduced with oxprenolol before slow and rapid fire (Fig. 1; Table 1). The reduction in heart rate was confirmed in those volunteers with continuous electrocardiographic recording. Both the maximum heart rate attained and the frequency peak were reduced with oxprenolol.

Blood samples were not obtained from all subjects. In the slow-fire study, mean free fatty acid levels were lower with oxprenolol as compared to placebo. Cholesterol levels were significantly lower with oxprenolol 40 mg but not 80 mg. There were no significant differences in triglyceride, low-density lipoprotein (LDL) and plasma catecholamine levels between the oxprenolol-treated and the placebo groups. Side effects were as common with placebo as with oxprenolol.

Thus, single oral doses of oxprenolol taken before slow-fire pistol shooting produced significant improvements in target scores (Table 2). It was surprising that oxprenolol taken before rapid-fire pistol shooting did not. It was thought that rapid fire would be more stressful than slow fire, but it seems that the tension generated during slow fire is greater. A similar reduction in heart rate was obtained in the two studies, indicating similar activity. James (1977) found a reduction in tremor with oxprenolol, which may account for the improved scores during slow fire. During short bursts of rapid fire there may be less time to develop sufficient tremor to impair performance.

Scores were not consistently reduced on oxprenolol, confirming that low doses of oxprenolol do not impair central nervous function. Subjects taking oxprenolol consistently reported improved concentration and well-being during shooting and nervousness was reduced. The improvement in target scores tended to be more marked in those with low scores. These subjects also tended to have a higher heart rate, indicating greater anxiety. This study demonstrated that low doses of oxprenolol reduce emotional and physiological responses to stress without impairing the performance of a skilled task (accurate pistol shooting).

As a direct result of stress, rises in heart rate, systolic pressure and free fatty acid levels may damage the cardiovascular system. It would seem reasonable to protect the system by giving oxprenolol to subjects at risk. This may be beneficial in the long term by preventing the development of cardiovascular disease in healthy subjects.

Reference

James, I. M., Pearson, R. M., Griffith, D. N. W. and Newbury, P. (1977). Effect of oxprenolol on stage-fright in musicians. *Lancet* **2**, 952.

Heart Rates of Surgeons During Operating and their Modification by Oxprenolol
(Abstract)

G. E. FOSTER

Nottingham General Hospital

We have monitored the heart rates of surgeons engaged in operating and have shown that during operations the mean heart rate for a group of 8 surgeons was 121/min with peaks up to 150/min and over. When these surgeons were taking busy outpatient clinics their mean heart rate was 94/min. Tachycardia during operating was completely abolished by oxprenolol 40 mg, the mean heart rate for the group falling to 84/min ($P < 0.001$) (Fig. 1).

We then carried out a prospective randomized controlled trial during which a group of surgeons took oxprenolol 40 mg or a matching placebo before 4 operating lists. An assessment of surgical performance was made during each list by means of 3 tests assessing suturing accuracy, tremor, and concentration and reaction time. Heart rates were again reduced by the oxprenolol from a mean of 127/min to 83/min and there was no difference between the placebo and oxprenolol groups for any of the performance tests. Subjective feeling assessed on a visual analogue scale were not affected by either preparation, but surgeons were surprisingly unaware that they had taken oxprenolol.

Whatever the relevance of surgeons' tachycardia

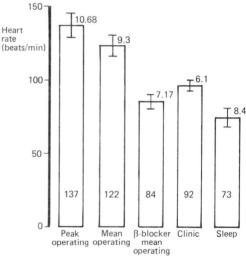

Figure 1. Mean heart rates of all subjects at peak operating, mean operating, mean operating under beta-blockade, while taking a clinic, and during sleep.

to development of ischaemic heart disease and life expectancy, their survival is considerably better than that of general practitioners (Table 1).

Table 1
Deaths among general practitioners and surgeons as a percentage of expected deaths

	Death (all causes)		Death (ischaemic heart disease)	
	No. observed	% of expected	No. observed	% of expected
General practitioners	2589	109[a]	1066	114[b]
Surgeons	679	86[a]	235	76[b]

[a] $P < 0.001$. [b] $P < 0.001$.

The Cardiovascular, Metabolic and Psychological Interface: Royal Society of Medicine International Congress and Symposium Series No. 14, published jointly by Academic Press Inc. (London) Ltd., and the Royal Society of Medicine.

Discussion
J. P. O'Loughlin

One possible factor in this disparity in death rates between general practitioners and surgeons is that surgeons on the whole retire at 65, while some general practitioners may not retire until about 80. This would certainly load the figures against the general practitioners dying of ischaemic heart disease.

G. E. Foster

This is quite true. I do not think the figures take that into account but nevertheless the difference shown is altogether too striking to dismiss.

N. Oakley

I have had experience of competitive rifle-shooting and it did not surprise me in the least to hear that the effect of oxprenolol on slow-fire shooting was better than on rapid fire. I think in pistol-shooting particularly, as in my own field of rifle-shooting, it would be very intesteing to know the actual time aim was held during oxprenolol treatment and with placebo, rather than the score, which is dependent on many other factors. Were any measurements made of this?

L. C. Antal

No, we did not measure differences in time aim was held but since subjects taking oxprenolol had less tremor, they probably held their aim longer.

P. G. F. Nixon

It is reasonable to regard well practised pistol-shooting as analogous to musicians playing well rehearsed pieces, which is largely under subcortical control. This type of performance can be improved by the abatement of somatic tremor, but I do not accept that these results can be extrapolated to the cortical function of handling new and complex information at speed, neither do I think the study would satisfy the Institute of Aviation Medicine that beta-blockade is free enough from adverse effects on flying, or driving ability, to use safely. In the study on surgeons, stressful operations were specifically excluded so that the surgeon was unlikely to be confronted by the problem of handling information which was novel or presented too rapidly. Why was cortical performance omitted from this carefully staged study which claims that the beta-blocker has some form of advantage for "performance" without the nature of the performance being specified?

G. E. Foster

I thought it would be fair to exclude the very difficult case in which the course of events can be unpredictable, but you can take it from me that even the average cholecystectomy can present all the difficulties in the world, and a fair few of these cropped up in this particular series.

P. G. F. Nixon

You were anxious lest these were adverse effects on that performance which you call stressful?

G. E. Foster

In our 2 trials we have not been able to show that either taking a beta-blocker or not taking it had any adverse effect on performance.

P. G. F. Nixon

Then why did you exclude the more complicated operations?

G. E. Foster

Because they are not perhaps as frequent as the other cases.

L. C. Antal

In our study we did actually seek the most stressful situation possible because we wanted to make sure that all those who took part had a very important goal ahead of them. In fact the results of our trials were so close that 2 more trials were needed before the team could be selected, so our subjects were under real stress. I would not agree that pistol-shooting is an entirely subcortical function; in fact, it is very much a cortical function.

N. Oakley

I must come in here. I do not know how much experience Dr Nixon has of competitive shooting and I think it is very dangerous for people to talk on a subject of which they have no knowledge. Twenty years ago I was lucky enough to win the gold medal in the World Rifle Championships in Moscow, and I am quite certain from my own considerable experience that the degree of coordination and of assessment of sophisticated interrelated variables involved in competitive rifle-shooting up to world standard is far from being subcortical.

P. J. Bourdillon

I was most interested in Dr Antal's study but I was rather concerned about the analysis of the data. When the frequency distribution curve is sigmoid in shape and the data scattered around the 50% mark, then normal statistical methods can be applied but at either extreme they lie on a very gradual slope and normal statistical methods are no longer valid. Did you use a logit or some other transformation before you worked out the statistics?

L. C. Antal

From a comparison of mean target scores for oxprenolol-takers and placebo-takers, both individually and as groups, it was clear that a large majority showed improvement in performance and there was no doubt in my mind that this was due to drug effect. As I said earlier, it was important that we chose subjects likely to be able to perform within a very narrow range of efficiency. Then variations in results would be due to drug effect rather than to individual effect or weekend effect, and so on. I think this has been demonstrated.

H. Keen

As I understand it, one of the recommendations for prophylaxis against coronary heart disease is to take daily exercise which accelerates the pulse rate to 120 beats/min or so. Do you suppose this might be the explanation for the unexpectedly better survival rates of surgeons compared with GPs?

May I couple with that a question on the effects of high body weight? If an individual is carrying a fat load around with him, he is continuously subjecting himself to an exercise load. Could this account for the fact that minimal mortality, both total and cardiovascular, occurs at something like +120% of so-called ideal body weight?

G. E. Foster

I should have thought that the rises in heart rate to which you referred were dangerous because they are taking place under conditions of relative inactivity, as in the case of public speakers and airline pilots, whose blood lipid levels are known to rise under these circumstances.

H. Keen

It could also be argued that a rise in blood fatty acid levels means that lipids are being mobilized and these could include deposits in the arterial wall.

G. E. Foster

But they are being mobilized in preparation for the fight-or-flight reaction which later is not made.

H. Keen

That may just be a myth. In fact, if we look at the survival rate in surgeons, as I understand it they do rather better than expected in the general population, and considerably better than general practitioners.

S. H. Taylor

The answer may depend on whether general practitioners, who appear to have a greater risk of coronary heart disease than hospital doctors, show the same cardiac responses to the stress of their occupation. Some years ago we examined the heart rate in vascular surgeons during operation and found a similar order of tachycardia to that described by Dr Foster, but we also found a similar tachycardia in many general practitioners during their surgeries, particularly if the patient load was heavy. We also found little tachycardia in hospital consultants during outpatient clinics. In all instances, oxprenolol 40 mg taken one hour before significantly reduced the tachycardia. If the tachycardia does indeed indicate the level of mental stress, then the different responses of consultants and practitioners may reflect different abilities to cope with the unexpected. These cardiac reactions are interesting but, however attractive the concept, we have insufficient data to extrapolate the relationship to one of cause (mental stress—tachycardia) and effect (coronary heart disease).